Pharmacodynamics in Spagyric Medicine

(Plant Alchemy)

By

Dr. Debasish Kundu

M.D.H., F.F.Hom, F.I.H.M.S., Ph.D. (U.S.A.), D.Sc. (Colombo)

&

Dr. Sudeshna Kundu

M.D.H. (U.S.A.), C.G.O. (Mumbai), M.F.Hom. (U.S.A.)

Edited By

Gisela Brueckl Ph.D.

and

El Akrem Hayouni Ph.D.

Foreworded By

Peter Morrell

B.Sc., PGCE, M.Phil.(London)

PUBLISHING

First Published 2017

Illustrations: Authors

ISBN 978-0-9993122-1-6

Published by
LBO Publishing
700 N Valley St., Suite B PMB 11884
Anaheim, CA 92801, USA
e-mail: info@LBOpub.com

In association with
Originals
A-6, 2nd Floor, Nimri Commercial Centre,
Ashok Vihar Phase 4, Delhi 110052 (INDIA)
e-mail: info@LPPindia.com

Printed and bound in India at:
Monica Enterprises
Delhi (India)

Prof. Dr. Debasish Kundu

M.D.H., F.F.Hom, F.I.H.M.S., Ph.D.(U.S.A.), D.Sc.(Colombo)

Fellow of International Holistic Medical Society, CA, U.S.A.

Fellow of Foundation of Homeopathy, MO, U.S.A.

Fellow of World E.Homeopathy System of Medical Council, Hong Kong

Faculty, International Holistic Medical Society, CA, U.S.A.

Faculty, Association of Independent Natural Science Schools Colleges, Professions & Arts, MO, U.S.A.

Vice-President, American Nutritional Medical Association, CA, U.S.A.

Foreign Bureau Chief (India), Holistic Medical Hylite International, CA, U.S.A.

Visiting Professor, Khulna Homeopathic Medical College & Hospital, Khulna, Bangladesh

Ex-Director General, Mooreland University, U.S.A.

Former Adjunct. Faculty & Associate Professor, Department of Human Behavior, Newport University, U.S.A.

Editor In Chief, International Journal of Homeopathy & Natural Medicines, USA

Editor in Chief, The Internet Journal of Herbal and Plant Medicine, USA

Author,

Diseases of Women,

Natural Medicines,

A Clinical Treatise on Cancer,

Aids & Homeopathy,

Pharmacodynamics,

Aids & Your Sex Life,

Aids & Homeopathy,

Essentials of Acupuncture,

Materia Medica for the New Age Man, etc.

Recipient, Royal Assyrian Order of Merit (OIUCM, 1993)

Laureate, United Nations Dag Hammarskjold Award for Medicine (1995)

Recipient, Special Achievement Award, International Conference on E. Omeopatia, Poretta Terme, Bologna, Italy (2008)

Dr. Sudeshna Kundu

M.D.H., C.G.O. (Mumbai), M.F.Hom (U.S.A.)

Member, Board of Governors, International Homeopathic Medical Society, CA, USA

Member, American Foundation for Homeopathy, MO, USA

Author,

Inimicals & Antidotals in Homeopathy, etc.

Gisela Brueckl

Ph.D., Pharmacist

Pharmacist, Adler-Apotheke Inh., Würzburg, Germany, Director General for Europe, American Nutritional Medical Association, CA, U.S.A.

El Akrem Hayouni

M.Sc., Ph.D.

Visiting Professor, High Institute of Biotechnology, University of Manouba, Tunisia

Visiting Professor, Faculty of Pharmacy, University of Monastir, Tunisia

Formerly Visiting Professor of Molecular Biosciences, TRBC, University of Ryukyus, Okinawa-Japan.

Peter Morrell

M.Sc., Ph.D.

Formerly Honorary Research Associate, History of Medicine, Staffordshire University, U.K.,

Author,

Hahnemann and Homeopathy,

Hahnemann's Homeopathy, etc.

Foreword

This book presents an excellent modern introduction to the ancient tradition of spagyric medicine. Some spagyric methods and concepts are clearly visible in Steiner's formulation of Anthroposophical Medicine, yet the term and its methods fell into disuse and have been rendered invisible for the last five centuries. This book therefore illuminates a largely forgotten area of medical history and medical practice. Spagyric medicine has been mostly associated with the names of Paracelsus and Van Helmont, who assembled the system from ancient fragments. Such methods of drug identification and preparation, in the European tradition, probably stretch back to the ancient Egyptians. Yet such medical systems were also active in ancient China and India, for example, pointing to an even more ancient confluence of pharmaceutical ideas and methods, and thus a more universal basis for spagyric drug preparation methods.

The Spagyric system does not come down to us bereft of an underpinning philosophy or set of fundamental principles. Along with the methods, these principles feature heavily in this uniquely insightful book. The reader will also find here a helpful glossary of equipment, terms, formulae (recipes) and symbols along with several useful methodologies of those key figures (such as Mattei, Zimpel, Krauss, et al) who rescued it from lost fragments and who thus played a major role in the recovery, development, preservation and exposition of spagyric principles and methods. Like a secret river flowing in darkness, spagyric medicine has been ignored and neglected for too long. This book serves to rekindle in the modern world an interest in the timeless value of spagyric methods and principles.

Peter Morrell
B.Sc., PGCE, M.Phil
Formerly Honorary Research Associate,
History of Medicine, Staffordshire University, UK, 1998-2007

Foreword

This work covers the section of Alchemy in Plant in Medicine, that is the art of Spagyrism. It is believed that the process of preparing the medicinal plant extracts through spagyric way, gives to the extracts a particular force; and that indeed every such extract is able to transport a particular Vital-Cosmic-Energy linked to the particular information of that own type of plant, more easily and more deeply of any other plant extract of the same species, to living human, animal and vegetal tissues and cells.

The talent of the Authors have been not only to enter deeply in this subject, but also to use a didactic exposition so the arguments are easily understood. Dr. Debasish Kundu is a leader scientific writer in the field of several CAM (Alternative and Complementary Medicines). He has been also our guest in Italy, at the Alkemy Laboratories, in Viareggio town, near Florence, in Central Italy, for learning ancient Italian-European Spagyric and Alkemic methodologies, and also for reciprocal teaching of Oriental-Indian techniques in the field in 2008.

So this book is a good introduction in Spagyric plant preparation.

Prof. Luigi Vernacchia
Alkeast Laboratories
Viareggio, VCarducci 55049,
Italia

Dr. Fabio R. Ambrosi N.D.
Lecturer, University of Sapienza,
Rome, Italia
Former Director,
Deptt. of Natural Medicines,
Universita Internazionale della
Nuova Medicina, Milano, Italia

Preface

Alchemy is the science of transforming and purifying substances providing insights into psychology, the inner archetypal structure of human thinking and feeling. Plant Alchemy is a type of mysticism in which alchemical transformation of plant materials are explored with mystical experiences. Alchemy gave impulses toward the preparation of medicinal remedies (mainly essential oils, plant extracts and essences) and considered the precursor science for pharmacology.

The preparation of alchemical or spagyric remedies is an ancient art of Indian origin. Gems are often used in Vedic astrology to mitigate negative influences of planets on human being. Philosopher's stone (cintamani) is one of the goals of alchemy. The name "alchemy" is derived from the arabic el-kimya, khem being the name for Egypt where it was practiced even before the Christian era. It blended with the magic and mysticism of the legendary Hermes Trismegistus which became known as the Hermetic philosophy.

In the fourth century A.D. alchemy evolved to its historical form. Its tradition reached Europe through Muslim alchemists in Spain in the twelfth century. Medieval alchemy contained Gnostic elements. In its popularized form it is considered the art of mutation of metals. Yet, it went deeper than that. It issued from the assumption that matter is alive and may grow. With the right rituals matter could be influenced to transmute into higher forms. Under the cover of semi-scientific experiments its practitioners followed a secret tradition. Thus, in its mystical sense alchemy was not a search for the philosopher's stone for the transmutation of metals into gold. Its deeper aspect was the search for purification of the soul, the mystical transmutation of the mind necessary for obtaining direct divine knowledge Cupellation of gold and silver which is an essential process in Alchemy, which is claimed to have been discovered by the Arabs, was known to the Siddhars (practitioners of Siddha System of Medicine) long before. Siddha Alchemy is older than Arabic Alchemy (850 BC to about 1500 AD) and Chinese Alchemy (300 BC to today). The Siddhars were also aware of several alchemical operations divided into several processes such as – calcinations, sublimation, distillation, fusion, separation conjunction or combination, congelation, cibation, fermentation, exaltation *i.e.* the action or process of refining gold, fixation, *i.e.* bringing to the condition of being non-volatile, *i.e.* to the state of resisting the action of fire, purification, incineration of metals, liquifaction, extraction and so on.

Siddha medicine is one of the oldest medical traditions too often confused with ayurveda, the ancient Indian science of life and health. It is a distinct branch of Ayurveda that started in southern India much before the Aryan era. Ever since the time of the legendary Sage Agastya and his 18 siddhars the ancient propagators and practitioners of this system Siddha knowledge has continued to percolate from master to disciple. Siddha System of Medicine is as old as mankind and dominated the civilisation of the southern peninsula of India. This civilisation dates back to 12,000 years before Christ. The findings of historians and the Tamil literary works such as "Tholkapiam," "Thiruvasagam" etc., reveal that there were three Tamil Academies for the growth of 64 Arts of Tamilians. The first Academy was in the old city of Madurai from 1990 BC to 5550 BC in the Tamilian continent called Lamuria, which comprised forty-nine districts to the south of cape comorin (India). There were 549 members in the Academy. Their code book was 'Agathiyam'. The Second Academy was held in the city of Kavadapuram 5550 BC to 1850 BC. During the King Mudu Thirumaran the Tamil Land was submerged in the sea. The king escaped from the sea deluge in a big ship and established the Third Academy in the modern city Madurai and lasted for about 1850 years. A number of Siddhars had representation in these three Tamil Academies. Among them were 18 Siddhars *viz.*, "Agasthiar, Bohar, Korakkar, Sivaya Siddar, Sattai Muni, Thirumoolar, Nandhi,

Koonakannar, Konganar, Manchamuni, Kalanginathar, Pathanjali, Kamalamuni, Idaikkadar, Punakeesar, Sundaranandar, Chandikesar, and Therayar" who contributed thousands of volumes on Siddha Medicine and imparted their knowledge through Guru-Sishya (master to disciple) principle.

The word Siddha comes from the word Siddhi which means an object to attain perfection or heavenly bliss,one of the fundamentals of Siddha methodology are Vadham which means Alchemy. According to Siddha medical science, the universe originally consisted of atoms which contributed to the five basic elements, *viz.*, earth, water, fire, air and sky which correspond to the five senses of the human body and they were the fundamentals of all the corporeal things in the world. The earth is the first element which gives fine shape to the body including bones, tissues, muscles, skin, hair, etc. Water is the second element representing blood, secretions of the glands, vital fluid, etc. Fire is the third element that gives motion, vigor and vitality to the body. It also helps digestion, circulation and simulation besides respiration and the nervous system. Above all, ether is the characteristic of man's mental and spiritual faculties.

This is also one of the basic principles of Ayurveda, Acupuncture and Alchemy. Alchemy is the medieval chemical science and speculative philosophy whose aims were the discovery of a universal cure for disease, and the discovery of a means of indefinitely prolonging life.

The alchemist believed all matter had a common origin and had the ability or potential to change shape, color, or appearance. The alchemist sought a complete scheme of things; in which God, the angels, man, animals, and the lifeless world all fitted into place. Also the origin of the world, its purpose, and end were to be clearly visible.

The term Alchemy, or "Al-Kemi", is said to be derived from Arabic or Egyptian meaning either "divine chemistry" or possibly "black earth" referring to the silt deposits from the annual flooding of the Nile river. However, regardless of where the word 'alchemy' began, it has come to mean a very special form of medical and spiritual development. Paracelsus (1493-1541) was the greatest physician of medieval times and an alchemist, he was the first in ascribing disease to "infectious seeds". He rejected previous medical views, believing that "like" cures "like". He concluded that the purpose of alchemy should not be to produce gold but to concoct medications to treat diseases. He had a profound impact on medicine and treatment of diseases.

Siddha generally refers to Athma Siddha that is the 8th supernatural power. The eight mighty Siddhic Process or Octo-Miracle ("Atta-Ma-Siddhi") which could keep the body strong and perfect for External Life, where there is no death or re-birth. Those who attained or achieved the above said powers are known as Siddhars. Siddha system of medicine is based on Saiva Siddhantha. who mostly worship their Lord Shiva as the Lingam or sacred Phallus, have had a difficult time accepting the Siddhas tendency to emphasize the Goddess. To the Siddhars, Shiva is the ultimate reality beyond form or comprehension, but Shakti, the Goddess, is immanent and accessible as the divine force abiding within the body itself. There she can be coaxed and subdued, manipulated and directed. As the serpent power Kundalini, flowing through the subtle body, she can propel the consciousness of the Siddhar into union with the Absolute. There the term is applied not only to one of the 18 categories of divine beings but also to Lord Shiva himself, who is a Siddha or Cittar because the very nature of God is consciousness. Likewise, it describes the devotee as also being a cittar since his consciousness is always immersed in the divine presence. By the 12th-13th century the term has taken on new meaning as we learn from the writings of Perumparrapuliyur Nambi who describes Lord Shiva as the cittar alchemist who is working strange miracles in the city of Madurai, South India, thus, Siddha is a tamil word that is derived from its root 'chit' which means perfection in life or "heavenly bliss".

Concurrently, Plant Alchemy is a timeless art because the basic principles, which align themselves to the phenomenology and natural laws of space and time, which never lose their validity. In the future, the importance of spagyric remedies will increase even further because their potency and effectiveness as a holistic medicine will not only be intuitively realised, but will also be proven in the same way that the interconnectedness of all life forms on the earth and in the cosmos is now being understood and proven. Spagyric Pharmacy, sometimes called Herbal Alchemy.

The spagyric art of producing a high quality medication is a method in which the transmutation patterns of plants, mineral and metallic substances that normally take place in nature as part of a larger evolutionary cycle, instead take place within a small laboratory setting, where they are quickened through the process of catalysis.

The word spagyric comes from the Greek word 'spao', which means separate, and ageirein, which means unify. A fundamental law of nature is that of polarity. This can be seen, for example, in the process of breathing: during inhalation, a part separates from the whole, and during exhalation the part again returns to the whole. There is an everchanging process of "dying and becoming", which, however, contains the dynamics of perfection.

The separation and unification processes used in the production of spagyric remedies should be seen as an attempt to increase the life energy found within a plant or mineral. This process of cohobation (elevation) is achieved through repeated distillations in which the distillate is repeatedly reunified with the residue, and the distillation is carried out a new.

Through continual changes in the aggregate conditions of the distillate and through the reunification with the residue in the distillation container, the distillate attains a high level of purity and, at the same time, its effectiveness is dynamised. Certain plants, minerals and metals each have their own specific distillation rhythm, and these are strictly observed. Depending upon the composition and/or structure of the particular mineral or plant needing to be "unlocked", either rhythmic distillations, also called rotations, or circulations, in which the distillations are carried out continually and repeatedly at constant temperature up to 33 times, are used.

The processes of solve and coagula that transpire during laboratory distillation not only refer to the separation and reunification of the distillate and the residue, but primarily refer to the separation of the plant, metal or mineral into the three active principles Mercury, Sulphur and Salt.

Mercury is the transpersonal spirit/mind principle. In a remedy, it is the carrier of information.

Sulphur is the soul principle. In a remedy, it represents the "personal" inner qualities and active ingredients within the substance. For example, in plants, these are the essential oils and aromas.

Salt is the physical principle. In a remedy, it includes the active ingredients that can be analysed, measured, weighed and even synthesized.

It should be clear that sulphur and mercury principles aren't found in synthetically produced remedies. In these types of remedies, only the physical level can be reproduced.

In homeopathy, the mercury principle is attained through the process of potentisation. In this case, it is the information within the substance that has been dynamised.

Hahnemann says in the Organon not to let the plant die; make the remedy from a live plant. He has a lot of requirements and directions that almost none of the pharmacies follow.

The preparation of spagyric essences is not always the same. There is no uniform method in the preparation as seen in homeopathy. And even the Philosophy may vary among the systems of spagyric methods.

In Spagyrics, there exist different systems: Of which the mains are the systems of Count Cesare Mattei (1809-1896), Dr. Carl-Friedrich Zimpel (1801-1879), Alexander von Bernus, Theodor Krauss (1864-1924), Dr. rer. nat. Peter Beyersdorff, Conrad Johann Glückselig (1864-1934) and Ulrich Jürgen Heinz.

Even though there are similarities in homeopathy and spagyrics, the roots of both systems being too different. Spagyric Homeopathy is a bridge between phytotherapy and homeopathy, in which micronutrients enriched plant essences are used to combat ailments.

Spagyric includes hermetic principles, rooting in ancient Egypt. In Europe, Paracelsus has been an important advocate of Spagyrics. Homeopathy came much later.

Spagyric is derived from "spao" = to separate, and "ageirein" = to combine. In spagyric remedy, larger organic molecules are not found anymore. So, poisoning by substances can not take place, even if poisonous plants are used. Spagyric production methods are holistic in every sense of the word. Because of this, their application has nothing to do with suppression, substitution or with the physiological emulation of disturbed life processes, as in the case for synthesized or standardized remedies. In spagyric remedies, information for both the repair and the reorganisation of disturbed regulatory systems are given simultaneously. The most important thing, however, is that the remedy supplies the patient with the life energy that he is lacking so that he can dynamically apply this core information and use regenerating building blocks toward an appropriate repair and re-synthesis.

In addition to this holistic therapy principle in spagyric medicine, the composition of the finished remedies, which are always mixtures, are composed of ingredients that are related to each other through function and or affinity to a particular organ.

For example, there is a holistic remedy specific to the liver and a composition that stimulates the eliminating function specific to the kidneys. These remedies are holistic in the sense that they act on all three levels of the human being and address his relationship to the surrounding cosmos.

All of the plants are dried on silk screens, and it is here, with these plants, that the beginning steps in spagyric production process take place. After observing the care and purity in which these spagyric remedies are prepared within our "toxic" world. Most diseases are the result of a loss of one's own inner biorhythm. People have forgotten that they are a microcosm within a macrocosm and that they are also affected by the natural cosmic and planetary rhythm. Indeed, we can only be healthy and whole when we are coherently attune to these rhythms.

Our immune systems as well as our metabolic processes are dependent upon rhythmic regulation. Every living system is in a rhythmic, vibrating state of balance. Health is a dynamic balance between chaos and order. Disease occurs there where the active rhythm between the poles has been lost. For this reason, a challenge for our day and age is to fundamentally turn away from the dead end street we are on, and to once again search for the true middle way.

The sun and moon, the two representatives of the polar rhythm of our being, compliment one another in a harmonious way –there can be no yin without yang, and no yang without yin. It is a gift to have remedies that contain within them the secret of the balance of energies and the structures that they form.

We dare to present this book before medical fraternity to unearth the timeless saga of Spagyric Medicine.

We are indebted to Dr. Vijay Kant Agnihotri, Scientist, CSIR, Dr. Mitchell Terry (U.K.), Dr. Peter Morrell (U.K.) and last but not the least eminent researchers of plant alchemy Prof. Luigi Vernacchia (Italy), and Dr. Fabio R.Ambrosi (Italy) for their valuable suggestions and support without which it could not be possible to complete this work.

Dr. Debasish Kundu
Dr. Sudeshna Kundu

Contents

Note to the Readers

No responsibility for loss or damage occasioned to any person acting, or refraining from action, as a result of the material in this publication can be accepted by the author.

Name of diseases are given in this book is for convenience only. The seat of the disease lies in the aberrance of some one or more of the constituents, which may be manifested in different forms, according to the constitution of the individual affected. Pathology, and a true reading of the meaning of the signs, or symptoms, of the disease, must be the guide to a true Spagyric prescription. Diseases bearing the same name vary as greatly as do the members of a family and something more than the correct classification of diseases, classification, is needed for a curative prescription.

Any information given in this book is not intended to be taken as a replacement for medical advice. Therefore, it is very important that the patients should avoid self-treatment and should consult with a specialist where appropriate.

Part 1

1

Introduction to Spagyric Medicine

Spagyric medicine is an ancient natural system of healing and has been brought up to date using modern pharmaceutical methods of manufacturing and safety standards.

The word "Spagyric" is coined from two Greek words meaning "to separate" and "to reunite", alluding to the specific preparation process of a Spagyric essence. During this process, the constituents of the plant will be separated, transformed, purified and recombined in modern laboratories by methods inspired by medical alchemy. The resulting Spagyric essence is natural, pure and possesses a full spectrum of healing properties for the entire human being. Derived entirely from plants, each individual spagyric essence is made from a particular plant, its healing power increased by Spagyric transformation. Given to a patient, such a remedy mobilises his/her self-healing forces.

Spagyric medicine is first attributed to Paracelsus, the great 16th century Swiss healer. Paracelsus was a healer, a physician and a professor of medicine. His teaching was widely discussed in most medical schools in Europe at the time and he is famed for his fight against orthodoxy as well as for his medical achievements. Paracelsus travelled widely to learn about other ways of healing. He brought medicine and alchemy together to create his own method. He strongly believed in the connection between humankind and nature and that plants were placed on Earth for our benefit. To Paracelsus is attributed the Doctrine of Signatures: the concept that the healing potential of a plant is shown in its very form, or "signature". Plants are natural remedies and their healing power can be increased by Spagyric transformation. But as per the information available in the Vedic texts which dates back to 7th century B.C. it was Agastya or Agasthyar who is considered to be the author of first Siddha literatures that includes writings in alchemy, medicine and spirituality.

Alchemy is a pretended science or art by which the metals are called base, such as lead and iron were supposed to be, but were never really, transmuted into the other metals as often called perfect, namely, gold and silver. The essence of Alchemy was pursued by many persons in the past, and though they did not succeed in making gold or silver, they yet unearthed through their scientific experiments many so called secrets of our world that they actually laid the foundations of chemistry as it is today. Some were the great chemists of their period.

The basic principal of Alchemy is that there are six basic kinds of elements available in this world. The whole world is made from combinations of these elements:

Magic

Magic is the root of most of the world, All other elements, except spirit, can be produced from magic with only an application of will (And the correct incantations of course). The use of magic seems to be dependant on the wielder having a base level of intelligence, and thus a stronger spirit than most animals although it has even observed that such base creatures such as goblins using magic, even though the chances of such creatures having entered any form of education is remote. Unfortunately in all cases, the presence of a skilled practitioner is always required. With Alchemical potions, a skilled practitioner is only required at the point of manufacture. This makes Alchemical potions a very practical backup to magicians and spiritualists when going in to dangerous locations, however not all magical effects can be duplicated using potions. However, there are also some potion effects such as powerful curing potions that are unavailable to magical practitioners.

Spirit

Spirit is the divine essence. It is what animates us. It is the Gods gift to the man that makes us aware of ourselves and others.

Everything living has some of this essence to some degree. Some people use the presence or absence of a spirit to define if something is truly dead.

The masters of the spiritual essence are of course the clerics to the various Gods, who have been given the ability to channel some of the divine essence at request, by their Gods.

Spirit can be harnessed in some small ways by the Alchemist, but there are some gifts given to clerics by their Gods that cannot be matched by mundane alchemical practices. However, there are again, some powers associated with Alchemy which are unavailable to clerics as well. Again the major advantage with Alchemy is that a skilled practitioner is only required at the point of production, not use.

Fire

Fire is the first of the base elements. It represents the destruction and change. Potions involving destruction and conversion tend to be very heavy in fire ingredients. These include ignite potions, poisons, and to a lesser extent, light potions.

Wind

Wind represents soothing, cooling and dissipation.

Potions which need to only last a small amount of time tend to have a heavy wind bias.

These include flash potions used to temporarily stun creatures.

Water

Water represents soothing and absorption.

Potions which need to be absorbed into materials tend to have a heavy water bias. These include curing balms, and potions intended for ingestion.

Earth

Earth represents permanence.

Potions which have a heavy earth bias include any potions intended for slow release, or potions which are used to form permanent items. It may be noted that earth potions tend to be diametrically opposed to fire biased potions because the fire is decidedly in- permanent and will consume the earth part of the material.

However, the correct balance of Earth and Fire can produce reasonably long lasting potions, for example, the difference between a light potion and a flash potion, is the balance. If the potion has more of the fire element, it burns brighter, If it has more of the earth element, it burns dimmer, but for longer.

All the materials in our world are a fundamental balance of the six elements. Most materials commonly found are a mixture of the four lesser elements. Magical essence is rarely found in any natural form, and Spiritual essence quickly leaves any material that is dead (another reason to use fresh ingredients, herbs to be specific).

Without using pure magic, it is very difficult to directly modify the balance of elements within a given material (actually, even with magic, it is not a trivial feat, at least not in a controllable manner). Therefore to achieve the correct balance of essences, materials containing other balances must be mixed in precisely measured quantities, and using precise methods to release these essences into a more useful form. The skilled use of these methods is what separates the Alchemist from the common pharmacist.

Astrology

Astrology is likely one of the most misunderstood aspects of esoteric philosophy, often seen as mere fortune telling. In reality, astrology- like the other aspects of the Organic Unity paradigm, is based on direct observation of nature. Its roots go back to ancient Mesopotamia, and is considered the sister science to alchemy. Whether one believes in astrology or not, the fact remains that it has been a part of numerous cultures from around the world for thousands of years and that it works- regardless of the system used. Systems do not stick around for thousands of years if they lack validity. The two practical uses of astrology within this system are for the preparation of medicinal substances and for specific evaluation of ones health.

As for the preparation of plant medicines, astrology teaches about proper timing. Thus, the plant is able to be harvested, prepared, and utilized in a way that is harmonious with the plants own energetic constitution. For example, if one has a plant ruled by the Sun, it would be harvested and processed on Sunday at the

Sun hour, thus exalting that energetic component of the plant. This would make the remedy more specific for a person's own inner Sun, being the heart and overall vitality. Astrology allows for correspondences and connections to be made between a plant, a person, and the cosmos.

The connection between plants and planets can be seen etymologically, as they derive from the same root "plane." Plants and Planet, they are mirror images of one another, with one reflected in the sky and the other reflected on Earth. It was common practice for herbalist in the ancient times to have a thorough understanding of the stars in order to properly align their medicines with their celestial counterpart, as well as effectively diagnose and treat their patients. The natal chart can be used as a tool to understand the preconditioned strengths and weaknesses of ones being (constitution/temperament) and thus the energetic architecture that determines how and when they will get sick.

The three modes of astrology correspond with the three principles of alchemy, the three worlds of the Shaman, and the three doshas of Ayurveda. The four elements of astrology are the same within all of the systems. The seven planets are a more complex expression of the pattern of existence: Sun, Moon, Mercury, Mars, Venus, Saturn and Jupiter. Whereas the four elements provide the energetics of a particular season, the planets provide a more refined picture of the pattern at play in nature. The twelve archetypes or signs, give further specificity. Each level or dimension is a different lens of perception, and gives different layers of information.

The Organic Unity Paradigm

As a paradigm of healing, medicine making, and cosmology, Organic Unity pulls from various traditional systems worldwide mainly alchemy, herbalism, astrology, ayurveda, science and shamanism. By weaving these traditions together, a truly holistic understanding of self, nature, and the healing process may be achieved. Each system makes a unique contribution to understanding and one may fill in a gap that is present in another. This paradigm is truly holistic in the sense that it brings us into harmony with the wholeness of existence, from the most distant star, to the smallest molecule.

The world is a melting pot of information, and seeing the similarities and weaving together paradigms, traditions and cultures, helps us to understand where we come from, where we are going, and what is the healthiest way to move forward on this planet. It is our goal to assist in a positive shift in our paradigm to one that is harmonious with existence. It is our hope that this information may help you in some way on your path of understanding in creating positive change in the world.

A Spiritual Science

This paradigm is a map of nature and how to best come into harmony with it. But the map is not the terrain it is mapping, it is only a signpost; it helps to guide the way. Maps are useful tools to have, but if the focus is always on the map, the landscape will not be experienced directly. These various maps of ayurveda, alchemy, shamanism, astrology, etc. only provide different lenses to perceive the landscape of existence, but the goal is to come to a direct connection with existence. Truth never comes by studying it. Once a direct connection is established, it can be reflected upon with the map in order to understand where one is and how to best navigate. It is best understood as a spiritual science.

Cosmology

Each part of the Organic Unity contains a certain cosmology which gives insights into the architecture of the universe. Cosmology by definition is "the study of the universe in its totality and its origins." While this is one of the more controversial subjects among religions and science (which has become a religion unto itself), correspondences can be drawn when one begins to peer beyond the surface level of what is being said. Genesis can be related to big bang, which can be seen in the ayurvedic and alchemical cosmologies. After all, they are explaining the unfolding of the same universe, just from different points of perception and cultural conditionings.

Cosmology enables us to understand the patterns behind the material world and how they are put together and interact with each other. It shows the pattern of interconnectedness. Modern holographic theory states that within each part, the whole is reflected. Thus, one can see the entire universe within a plant, a person, or a cell, or anything. But what does this mean, and how it is useful? To the seeker of wisdom and healing, it is the most important thing to realize, because everything instantly becomes ones teacher and healer. The entirety of creation becomes the voice of the infinite one, the organic is an expression of the unity. We are no longer separate from the rest of creation, because we within ourselves contain all of creation. Thus by studying creation, we study ourselves.

Most cosmologies are energetic, meaning they are expressions of the invisible. When one is speaking of the building blocks of the universe, it is impossible to speak in terms of strict physicality and rationality. There is no one single molecule or atom that is the fundamental building block. Terrence McKenna opined that "science has pushed the boundary of the rational world far enough to see its irrational basis." Quantum physics has shown that when you get down to the smallest parts of matter, it starts to not look like matter anymore, but energy. Cosmology is the study of the energy that exists prior to matter, but is contained within matter. It is the space between the unseen and the seen, or how the invisible manifests into form.

The practical application of this knowledge is towards an understanding of ones own energy, ones own inner cosmology. This lends insight into the physical constitution, and the mental/emotional temperaments, along with their inherent strengths and weaknesses. From here, those weaknesses and imbalances can be strengthened and healed through the application of natural substances by understanding their own unique cosmology and how the two relate. This assists in the healing process of revealing ones true essential nature and life purpose.

One of the easiest ways to understand cosmology is through two of the most ancient sciences: numerology (sacred mathematics) and sacred geometry. These give the most simple and practical ways to see these energetic patterns. The whole universe can really be understood as various combinations of numbers.

It all starts from oneness, the infinite, when the universe existed in a state of pure potential. In geometry, it is the point. This oneness is the unity point from which the organic arises. It is from this point that all manifestations arise, and all things return to in their time. It is the Great Spirit, God, Allah- the one who is known by many names. It is important to remember, that each set of numbers are a reflection of the one, just in more complex form.

The one then divides into two, which is the principle duality- the masculine/feminine, day/night, Sun/Moon, Yang/Yin. This is the creation of the space/time continuum. Geometrically, the point becomes the line. These two forces interact and create the three, which is the trinity, or triangle. These are the three philosophical principles of Alchemy, the modes of Astrology, the doshas of Ayurveda.

From three it moves into the four, which is the square, the four winds or elements. Organic Unity works within a natural elemental system: Earth, Water, Fire, Air, and Ether being the invisible fifth element.

The other two main sets of harmonics of practical use are the seven and the twelve. These are the astrological patterns of the planets and the archetypes or signs. These provide the most specific and individualized reflections of the unity.

The Four Sacred Directions

Another aspect of the shamanic cosmology is the four sacred directions, or the four winds. These four sacred directions also correspond to the four natural elements (Earth, Water, Fire, Air), and depending on the tradition, tend to vary in their correlation. This has been called by some Earth astrology. The four directions are ways of connecting with the seasons of our lives, and understanding them greatly assists in coming into harmony with our own natural rhythms and patterns. It is a pattern of time cycles. Each direction typically has an animal, plant, or mineral that holds the energetic quality that corresponds to it, as well as different organ systems in the body. It also has a correlation to different cycles of time: day, year (season), and our entire life. One can meditate on these different seasons and cycles of time and come to greatly understand the energies of the directions.

The wheel typically begins in the East, the place of the rising sun, the dawn of a new day and the spring time. It is all about newness, fresh starts, and the shining of light in places where there was once darkness. Illumination and inspiration all fall in the east, as does the element of air and the bird tribes (Eagle, Hawk, Condor). In the East, we are able to gain a distant perspective on our lives, to see far into the future and understand what the best direction we are to take. We see things in the light of a new day. The East relates to childhood, adolescence, and correlates to the archetype of the teacher.

Next is the South: high noon, summer time, and the element of fire. It is here that we learn the art of celebration, innocence, and travel. We dance our dance, sing our song, and share our existence with others. In the East we have gained insight and understanding into our lives, in the South we share that understanding. It is here we learn the lessons of the heart: the full, clear, open and strong heart. Coyote lives there. The South relates to early adulthood and is correlated to the archetype of the visionary.

The West correlates to the dusk, autumn, and the element of water. It is in this place that we begin our journey inward to reflect on the expansiveness and extroversion of the East and South. The West is the looking within place, and is a time for looking into the patterns we carry that must be let go of in order to become who we truly are. This is the lesson of the autumn trees who drop their leaves to nourish the Earth once again. Bear and Crow reside in the West, along with all of our ancestors. This is usually a time of great emotion, slowing down, and gathering ourselves for the winter ahead. The West relates to adulthood/middle age and correlates to the archetype of the healer.

The final turn on the medicine wheel is the North: the night, winter, and the element of Earth. The North is the place of nothingness, where we return to the Great Mystery to receive our vision to be ignited in the East. It is a place of the three dreams: the day dream, the night dream and the life dream. This is the time where we are to dream deep and wide, for the vision of our life purpose and who we truly are. Deep ancient elders and wise ones live in the North, but we must be able to empty ourselves to receive their wisdom. It is the place of the Owl and other nocturnal animals. The North relates to elder-hood and correlates to the archetype of the warrior.

By understanding the energetic architecture of the seasons, times of day, and times of our lives, we can better come into harmony with it and integrate the lessons life is bringing our way. It also helps to correlate things that are seemingly disparate, as everything has a place on the wheel and is thus related to everything else. So, by understanding where a plant resides on the medicine wheel, certain correlations can be drawn to animals, seasons, and states of consciousness and experiences that would otherwise not be able to be related. It is a simple map that can be ones guide for life.

The Three Worlds of Shamanism

Within the shamanic cosmology, the world is divided into three levels: the upper, lower, and middle worlds. This is often symbolized by a world tree, with the roots, trunk, and branches corresponding to the lower, middle and upper worlds, respectively. This is the trinity of shamanism. Each level contains within it a certain vibrational quality that holds specific wisdom and healing that is accessible to the shaman by entering a non-ordinary or altered state of consciousness. The ability to enter the other reality is frequently achieved through the use of a drum, rattle, dancing, chanting, and medicinal plants or mushrooms. The shaman travels through these three worlds to gather information and medicines that are specific for the person they are working with.

The lower world is commonly misperceived as being the place where evil spirits live, darkness pervades, and in general, not a good place. This is mainly due to our cultural conditioning of hell being "down there", and heaven being "up there." The lower world is in fact the place where many spirits of nature reside. It is a place where the essence of a plant, mineral, animal, mountain, lake, or any other aspect of nature can be connected and communed with. In this way, the lower world provides information into nature, and the invisible web of interconnections that it contains. It is often a place where ones power animals reside, as well as plant totems. The lower world could also be considered microcosmically to be our unconscious of subconscious self, those parts of our being which are constantly at play but yet we are unaware of.

The middle world is our reality as we know it. It is our day to day lives and residing place of our physical bodies and our normal waking consciousness. The middle world reality is full of trials and tribulations, tests and blessings, yet it is only one third of the tree of life. If we are not rooted in the wisdom of the lower world, our trunk will not be able to carry the nourishment that the branches need to reach full flowering. In order for our middle world reality to be understandable, a firm groundedness in the underworld is necessary, that is, entering a communion with the invisible dynamics of nature, the spiritual essences of the natural world. The middle world would be considered our ego, or conscious self.

The upper world is what some call the "heavens." The is the home of the star nations, our celestial or spirit guides, the angels and archetypes (twelve astrological signs), and the planetary beings. Microcosmically, the upper world relates to our higher self, or superconsciousness that permeates across all time and space. The upper world is where we turn for spiritual guidance and wisdom that is of a higher vibrational quality than that of lower world wisdom. It is not better, just a different quality. The upper world reveals the depth of our true essential nature that will allow us to enter into the flowering of our purpose. It is our peak, our summit. It is here that we receive the guidance that will take us closer to being in harmony with the unity.

Each world is an absolutely necessary part of our own being and the universe at large. Neither has teachings or healings that are better or worse than the other- they are just different. This is why the analogy of a tree is so useful; we cannot say that the roots are worse than the flowers. Without those roots, the flowers would not be possible, and there must be a stem to connect the two. Each part has its place in the pattern of the whole, and yet, the whole cannot be recognizable by studying the parts. We cannot understand the whole of the tree by looking at the roots, then looking at the trunk, and then the flowers. We must step back and look at that tree as a whole organic being, only then can the depth of its being be experienced. So it is with our own beings. We must respect and honor all parts of ourselves and not get lost in living in any one of the worlds exclusively. We must become fluid rivers of consciousness that is able to flow between all worlds and states of consciousness with ease and acceptance, but not forgetting to step back and look at the unity.

Spagyric is a unique and harmonious blend of herbal medicine, homeopathy, aromatherapy and mineral therapy. Spagyric medicine focuses on the underlying causes of health problems, which are often linked with past emotional and psychological issues: it thus leads to a more holistic healing. This natural therapeutic system embraces both the ancient medical wisdom and the latest scientific knowledge. It is always evolving to meet the challenge of current health issues. Spagyric presents to modern practitioners a large variety of remedies for all facets of human ailments. In contrast with certain traditional plant remedies, Spagyric is totally non toxic and without known side effects.

Spagyric essences are made from plants by a unique process, which neutralises their toxic components, but preserves their healing potential. It is a concentrated essence, sometimes slightly coloured with typical flavours and smells. It is not recommended to dilute Spagyric essence, as unlike Homeopathy it is non-toxic and free from heavy metals or other potential impurities.

2

History of Alchemy

As per The Skeptic's Dictionary by Robert Todd Caroll, Alchemy is an occult art and pseudoscience. Its practitioners' main goals have been:

1. to turn base metals (like lead or copper) into precious metals (like gold or silver) (the transmutation motif);
2. to create an elixir or potion or metal which could cure all ills (the medical motif), and
3. discover an elixir which would lead to immortality (the transcendence motif).

The magical substance that was to transmute metals, to be the universal panacea and to serve as the key to immortality was called the philosopher's stone. Alchemy is based on the belief that there are four basic elements : fire, air, earth and water, and three essentials: salt, sulfur and mercury. Great symbolic and metaphysical systems have been built from these seven pillars of alchemy. The work of the alchemists provided the basis of modern laboratory techniques, and they unearthed many of nature's secrets. Their dogged pursuit for the elixir of life is not so different from modern chemists and natural products researchers who are similarly searching for that one great find which will cure all illnesses. In the mid-17th century, with the publication of Robert Boyle's The Sceptical Chymist, was there the beginning of a separation between alchemy and chemistry.

Indian Alchemy

History of Alchemy is applied to world's oldest medical science of India, Siddha Medicine. As per the information available in the Vedic texts it was Maharshi Agasthyar who is considered to be the author of the first Siddha literatures and he was supposed to have lived in the 7 th century BC. About 96 books are attributed to him and that includes writings in alchemy, medicine and spirituality. Agasthyar and his clan are also credited to have "authored" many mantras of the 7000 year old Rig Veda. Agasthyar is also the author of Agastya Samhita. Maharshi Agasthyar was the first to solidify mercury through the use of herbs. The Siddhas said to have consumed purified mercury, Iridium, Rhodium and gold in order to achieve physical immortality. The method of processing mercury for therapeutic purposes is known as Rasa Suthi in Siddha system of medicine. Siddhars used Mercury, by pulverising with rare herbal juices, using various amalgamation processes like impregnating and triturating with organic materials, etc., they are made homologous to the tissue cells and their toxicity is reduced and acceptability to the cell is increased. During this process certain organic and inorganic materials are also added. Mercury thus purified and processed is converted into healing nectar or amazing elixir, Gowri Chintamani, not only was used to cure innumerable diseases, but also to rejuvenate the body and promote longevity. In alchemy, the mercury rasa substitutes itself for human bodily fluids and thereby transforms a body of flesh and blood into a golden (swarna), adamantine (vajra), or perfected body (siddha) body. Agasthiyar, Thirumular and Bogar, three of the Siddhars in the lineage of the 18 Siddhars have contributed to the preparation of mercury laden Siddha medicines which can regenerate human cells. According to Siddha alchemy, Mercury is the representation of male (Shiva) form and the chemical element sulfur associated in the solidification process considered as the representation of female (Shakti or Gauri, consort of Shiva) form.

According to the Philosophy of Ancient Siddha Alchemy, the Eight Siddhis or attainments are:

1. Anima- Reducing one's body even to the size of an atom.
2. Mahima- Expanding one's body to an infinitely large size.
3. Garima- Becoming infinitely heavy.
4. Laghima- Becoming almost weightless.
5. Praapti- Having unrestricted access to all places.

6. Prakaamyam- Realizing whatever one desires.
7. Ishitvam- Possessing absolute lordship.
8. Vashitvam- The power to subjugate all.

ASHTA SIDDHI
EIGHT WAY POWERS

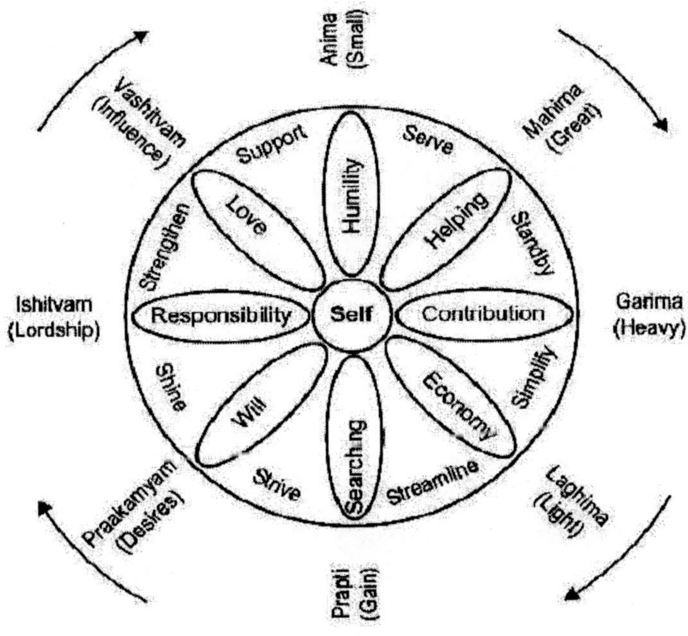

These are the eternal powers of ancient siddhars or alchemists of India.

All these can be attained by any one who strives, endeavours and does "Sadhana".

1. One can become small by being Humble. Humility can make us small. Let people underestimate us. Surrender, Stand under and understand. Practice of humility gives the power of "Anima".
2. One can become "Mahaan" the great, by helping others. Who ever serves others is Mahatma. Practice of helping others gives the power of "Mahima".

3. One can become heavy by the weight of one's contribution. Add value and become a heavy weight. Practice of continuous contributions can give the power of "Garima".
4. One can become light by shedding excess luggage, excess weight, wasteful practices and by shedding desires and ego. Economy and Egolessness give the power of "Laghima".
5. One can gain whatever one aspires by searching. Continuous search will lead to gain. Searching is Sadhana. Search and research for gaining the objective. Searching will lead to the power of "Praapti".
6. One can fulfil all desires through will power. Our will power is our "Kama Dhenu". If you will, you will. Will power can lead to the power of "Praakamyam".
7. One can become lord and leader by taking responsibility. A responsible leader is an effective leader. Responsibility can give the power of "Ishitvam".
8. One can influence all by love, care and concern. Caring can lead to the power of "Vashitvam".

These are eight powers or qualities required to be a perfect Alchemist according to Siddha philosophy and can be achieved through practice and persuasion. But desiring these powers as ultimate goals with personal wrong intentions, one will not achieve it.

Marco Polo came to Malabar, Kerala, India in 1293, and has made records of Siddha alchemy. He records a meeting he had with a group of alchemists who, by consuming a tincture consisting of Mercury and Sulfur, were afforded a lifespan of 50-200 years.

Ayurveda dates back to 3000 B.C., it has been said that there were Magha Bheshaja and Purohit (Magha Spagyric Ayurvedic practitioners and Priests) who are said to have cured the leprosy of Prince Samba, the son of Lord Sri Krishna in Mahabharata times. Magha physicians used to travel from one country to another to spread their knowledge. They are said to be originally from Sakyadwipa (probably Scythia). In those times, Iran was called as Madra (King Shalya and the Iranian Madri, the wife of Pandu was from Madra) and Greece was called as Ayoana which later became Yavan in classic Sanskrit and Ion in Persia. These Maghas were astronomers and physicians in Pre-Zoroastrian times in Persia and were called Maga or Mada in Persia. Maghas traveled to Greece and settled there. These Maghas used to cure the disease promptly with help of herbs and metals probably using the method of Spagyrism. The word Magha became Magus in Greek and Magis in Latin, and turned into the word Magic in old brythonic English.

This is the etymological history of word Magic which is related to alchemy. That is how the alchemical medicines used to be prepared on the herbal basis.

In the Rig Veda, written in Sanskrit, there are 117 hymns about a wonder elixir by the name of Soma. Soma Rasa was known as an exhilarating divine elixir.

The elixir itself was a hermaphrodite due to its compounded nature. That these elixirs were believed to be crucial to immortality is widely accepted within the history of the subject, but what is less understood is the mechanism of action by which they were supposed to work. What was the magic hiding within these elixirs that drove elixir-alchemists to attempt new elixir concoctions, or to be convinced of their potential for imparting immortality.

Some scholars say that Alchemy began in Greece and some say its root word comes from Egyptian root word Keme (Black), other says in Persian language the gold is called Khimiya but Indian Vedas throw a light on the history of Alchemy according to rasayan shastra, as India is the only nation that seems to be using the metals and herbal preparations down the centuries in different types of methods. Even soma rasa was prepared in pre-vedic times in India and "kim" the root word in Vedic Sanskrit means to transform. That's how it is related to Cheme of Chemistry or Alchemy. As Al is an Arabic prefix added to Chemiya, means that which transforms or transmutes.

Moreover in simple words, Alchemy means turning anything especially a material into a metal called gold and according to Ayurveda's Rasa Shastra which was one of the oldest Art of Vedic Alchemy, some ancient sages knew about its beneficial healing powers and were able to work on it successfully for medicinal purposes. Also, gold has many uses in Ayurvedic medical preparation. Rasa Sindoor is one product of Ayurveda where the curative properties (special efficacy as a medicine on the living body) of gold is transferred to a compound of mercury and sulfur where in the process gold that is used is measured at the end of process and in successful chemical processes it should by weighing as much as it was before the start of process.

The Chinese tried to make Siddha mercury elixir without proper understanding, the first emperor of China, Qín Sh Huáng Dì was killed by drinking a mercury and powdered jade mixture formulated by Qin alchemists (causing liver failure, mercury poisoning, and brain death). He got instant death instead of eternal life.

Indian word "Veda" means science or knowledge and "Rasaveda" means transforming a metal adding mercury oxide and transforming it into gold, so Alchemy was prevailing in India since the Vedic period.

Ulrich Arndt wrote on Alchemy and Ayurvedic Medicine in her article 'Seals of the Planets':

> "*Actually the secret Rubedo planet sequence* is known to everyone: It is encoded in the sequence of our weekdays' names and thus also in the Bible's Book of Genesis! As we know, the names of the seven weekdays are associated with the seven classical planets. The sequence of the following weekdays corresponds exactly to that third planet sequence.*"

Exactly the same correlation of planets and chakras as in the Rubedo sequence is known from the ancient Indian medicine of Ayurveda. Moreover, all the correlations of the seven metals and the seven most beneficial jewels with the planets – and so with the chakras – are identical in Alchemy and Ayurveda. Also in Ayurveda, certain colours are associated with the planets, and, strikingly, only the Rubedo planet sequence corresponds to the natural sequence of the rainbow. Furthermore, both medical systems employ the same means - specially formulated alchemistic essences of the seven metals and precious stones - to cure illnesses and to uplift a person's energy level. The spiritual effects of this chakra stimulation were also known in ancient India. For this reason, the jewel essences for the seven chakras were called "medicine of the Maharajas". For at least seven years they were administered to an heir apparent in order to prepare him emotionally and intellectually for his highest office. So, in a most impressive fashion, the medical and chakra teachings of Ayurveda corroborate the alchemistic developmental teachings about the three phases of transformation and the purpose of these teachings to guide humans, with every therapeutic intervention, towards the highest vibrational level of Rubedo.

Chakra Teachings of the Alchemists

Chakra	*Nigredo (Blackness)*	*Albedo I (Whiteness) Path of Contemplation*	*Albedo II (Whiteness) Path of the Heart*	*Rubedo (Redness)*
7. Crown chakra	*Saturn*	*Saturn*	*Sun*	*Saturn - Amethyst*
6. Forehead chakra	*Jupiter*	*Moon*	*Venus*	*Venus - Diamond*
5. Throat chakra	*Mars*	*Jupiter*	*Mars*	*Jupiter - Sapphire*
4. Heart chakra	*Sun*	*Mercury*	*Mercury*	*Mercury - Emerald*
3. Solar plexus chakra	*Venus*	*Mars*	*Jupiter*	*Mars - Yellow Topaz*
2. Spleen /sexual chakra	*Mercury*	*Venus*	*Moon*	*Moon - Pearl*
1. Root chakra	*Moon*	*Sun*	*Saturn*	*Sun - Ruby*
** Reddish-orange color of melting metals is referred to as Rubedo.*				

Chinese Alchemy

The founder of Chinese alchemy is considered to be Wei Po-Yang. Taoist monks pursued both the outer elixir and the inner elixir. The former being minerals, plants etc.

In the Eastern Han Dynasty, alchemists' thought of immortality developed into Taoism and alchemy became popular among ordinary people. Zhou Yi Can Tong Qi (A Comparative Study of the Zhou Dynasty Book of Changes) by Wei Boyang of the Eastern Han Dynasty is the earliest theoretic work on alchemy existing today in the world. The Inner Chapters of Baopuzi (The Master who embraces simplicity) by the Jin Dynasty alchemist Ge Hong documented and summarized the alchemy since the Han and Jin Dynasties in great detail.

References about alchemy are to be found in the myths and legends of ancient China. From a book written by Edward Chalmers Werner, a late member of the Chinese Government's Historiological Bureau in Peking comes this quotation from old Chinese records: "Chang Tao-Ling, the first Taoist pope, was born in A.D. 35 in the reign of the Emperor Kuang Wu Ti of the Han dynasty. Elixir Pills (Eastern Jin Dynasty; Unearthed from Tomb No. 7, Elephant Mountain in northern suburbs of Nanjing; Diameter: 0.5cm; Total Number: over 100 pills; Now preserved in Museum of Medical History, Shanghai University of Traditional Chinese Medicine)

Egyptian Alchemy

In ancient Egypt, where the word Khem was used in reference to the fertility of the flood plains around the Nile. Egyptian believed in life after death, and the mummification procedures they developed, probably gave rise to rudimentary chemical knowledge and a goal of immortality. When Egypt was occupied by the Arabs in the 7th Century, they added 'Al-' to the word Khem and Al-Khemia meaning 'the Black Land' is being told as the origin for the word alchemy. The great Egyptian adept king, named by the Greeks "Hermes Trismegistus" is thought to have been the founder of the art. Reputed to have lived about 1900 B.C., he was highly celebrated for his wisdom and skill in the operation of nature, but of the works attributed to him only a few fragments escaped the destroying hand of the Emperor Diocletian in the third century A.D. The main surviving documents attributed to him are the Emerald Tablet, the Asclepian Dialogues, and the Divine Pymander. If we may conclude from these fragments (both preserved in the Latin by Fianus and translated into other languages in the sixteenth century), it would seem to be of inestimable loss to the world that none of these works have survived in their entirety.

The famous Emerald Tablet (Tabula Smaragdina) of Hermes is the primary document of alchemy. There have been various stories of the origin of the tract, one being that the original emerald slab upon which the precepts were said to be inscribed in Phoenician characters was discovered in the tomb of Hermes by Alexander the Great. In the Berne edition (1545) of the Summa Perfectionis, the Latin version is printed under the heading: "The Emerald Tables of Hermes the Thrice Great Concerning Chymistry, translator unknown. The words of the secrets of Hermes, which were written on the Tablet of Emerald found between his hands in a dark cave wherein his body was discovered buried." An Arabic version of the text was discovered in a work ascribed to Jabir, which was probably made about the ninth century.

Arabian Alchemy

An Arabic version of the text was discovered in a work ascribed to Jabir Ibn Hayyan (8th century), which is regarded as the genuine Egyptian sacred art of alchemy. Jabir transformed alchemy through his use of scientific methodology and investigation. Instead of writing in coded words and phrases, Jabir was very straight forward in reporting his activities. In fact, he did not think alchemy was worth pursuing without experimentation. He was even willing to accept that it might be possible to create artificial human life in the laboratory. Jabir extracted anesthetic compounds from herbs, which were used for general anesthesia during operations or difficult procedures. He is also noteworthy for his introduction of a rudimentary elements system which eventually grew, over the centuries, into the table of elements we are familiar with today.

The third century A.D. seems to have been a period when alchemy was widely practiced, but it was also during this century, in the year 296, that Diocletian sought out and burnt all the Egyptian books on alchemy and the other Hermetic sciences, and in so doing destroyed all evidence of any progress made up to that date. In the fourth century, Zosimus the Panopolite wrote his treatise on The Divine Art of Making Gold and Silver, and in the fifth Morienus, a hermit of Rome, left his native city and set out to seek the sage Adfar, a solitary adept whose fame had reached him from Alexandria. Morienus found him, and after gaining his confidence became his disciple. After the death of his patron, Morienus came into touch with King Calid, and a very attractive work purporting to be a dialogue between himself and the king is still extant under the name of Morienus. In this century, Cedrennus also appeared, a magician who professed alchemy.

The next name of note, that of Geber, occurs in or about 750 A.D. Geber's real name was Abou Moussah Djfar-Al Sell, or simply "The Wise One." Born at Houran in Mesopotamia, he is generally esteemed by adepts as the greatest of them all after Hermes. Of the treatises composed by him, three remain to posterity: The Sum of the Perfect Magistery, The Investigation of Perfection, and his Testament. It is to him, too, that we are indebted for the first mention of such important compounds as corrosive sublimate, red oxide of mercury, and nitrate of silver. Skillfully indeed did Geber veil his discoveries, with great acuteness and precision.

An 11th-century Persian chemist and physician named Abû Rayhân Bîrûnî wrote,

"They have a science similar to alchemy which is quite peculiar to them. They call it Rasâyana, a word composed with rasa, i.e., gold. It means an art which is restricted to certain operations, drugs, and compound medicines, most of which are taken from plants.

Its principles restore the health of those who were ill beyond hope, and give back youth to fading old age."[*Alberuni's India*, transl. p. 188, Edward C. Sachau, vol. 1, London: Trübner and Co., Ludgate Hill, 1888.] Raseœvara, a school of Indian philosophy was focused on finding Moksha: perfection, immortality, liberation using mercury. As such it focuses its efforts on transumation of the human body: from mortal to immortal.

Many are the traditional stories of alchemists still alive since time immemorial due to the effects of their experiments. The texts of Ayurvedic Medicine and Science have aspects similar to alchemy: concepts of cures for all known diseases, and treatments that focus on anointing the body with oils.

Since alchemy eventually became engrained in the vast field of Indian erudition, influences from other metaphysical and philosophical doctrines such as Samkhya, Yoga, Vaisheshika and

Ayurveda were inevitable. Nonetheless, most of the Rasayâna texts track their origins back to Kaula tantric schools associated to the teachings of the personality of Matsyendranatha and the lineage of the Natha Siddhas.

Two famous examples were Nagarjuna and Nityanadhiya. Nagarjuna was a Buddhist monk who, in ancient times, ran the great university of Nagarjuna Sagara. His famous book, *Rasaratanakaram*, is a famous example of early Indian medicine. In traditional Indian medicinal terminology "rasa" translates as "mercury" and Nagarjuna was said to have developed a method to convert the mercury into gold.

About the same time, Rhasis, another Arabian alchemist, became famous for his practical displays in the art of transmutation of base metals into gold. In the tenth century, Alfarabi enjoyed the reputation of being the most learned man of his age, and still another great alchemist of that century was Avicenna, whose real name was Ebu Cinna. Born at Bokara in 980 A.D., he was the last of the Egyptian alchemical philosophers of repute.

European Alchemy

The introduction of alchemy to the west came in the 8th Century when the Arabs brought it to Spain., where it had been introduced by the Arabian Moors. The first European text to mention alchemy appeared roughly in 1050 CE. In the twelfth Century Artephius wrote The Art of Prolonging Human Life and is reported to have lived throughout a period of one thousand years.

Of the thirteenth century literature, a work called Tesero was attributed to Alphonso, the King of Castile, in 1272. William de Loris wrote 'Le Roman de Rose' in 1282, assisted by Jean de Meung, who also wrote 'The Remonstrance of Nature to the Wandering Alchemist' and 'The Reply of the Alchemist to Nature'. Peter d'Apona, born near Padua in 1250, wrote several books on Hermetic sciences.

The authority of Albertus Magnus (1234-1314) is undoubtedly unquestionable, he devoted the greater part of his life towards the study of alchemical philosophy and in the art of transmutation.

Raymond Lully born in Majorca about the year 1235, he traveled widely, not only in Europe, but in Asia and Africa, he is said to have become acquainted with the hermetic science. Records state that he lived to be one hundred and fifty years of age and was eventually killed by the Saracens in Asia. At that age he is reputed to have been able to run and jump like a young man.

During the fourteenth century, Acts of Parliament were passed in England to forbid the practice of alchemy. Although Pope John XXII is said to have practiced the art. Also, during this period the Isaacs Hollandus, the father and son duo, wrote three treatises, 'Opus Vegetabile', 'De Triplici Ordinari Exiliris et Lapidis Theoria' and 'Mineralia Opera Sue de Lapide Philosophico', in which a vivid account of most explicit details of their operations on plants and metals were given.

The beginning of the sixteenth century was characterized by publication of an important book: the Liber de arte de distillandi simplicibus due to Hieronymus Brunschwig (1450-1513), which appeared in 1500. This author, who we can consider the first precursor of Science Spagyric was to obtain the medicinal plants essential principles of distilling the water, or the macerate essential through a rudimentary steam stripping process.

The British Alchemists

Roger Bacon of England, a 13th century Franciscan Friar, who is considered one of the earliest proponents of the scientific method, is considered the first real European alchemist. Roger Bacon made many scientific discoveries. He was almost the only astronomer of his time, and in this capacity rectified the Julian calendar. Among his many writings, there are two or three works on alchemy, from which it is quite evident that not only he studied and practiced the science but that he obtained the final objective, the Philosopher's Stone. Sir George Ripley, Canon of Bridlington Cathedral in Yorkshire, placed alchemy on a higher level, he also worked on spiritual alchemy. He maintained that alchemy is concerned with the mode of our spirit's return to the God who gave it to us. His work 'Compound of Alchemy' was published in 1471.

Pierce the Black Monk in the sixteenth century, wrote: "Take earth of Earth, Earth's Mother (Water of Earth), Fire of Earth, and Water of the Wood. These are to lie together and then be parted. Alchemical gold is made of three pure soul, as purged as crystal. Body, seat, and spirit grow into a Stone, wherein there is no corruption. This is to be cast on Mercury and it shall become most worthy gold."

Thomas Charnock published a memorandum in 1572 in which he states that he attained the transmuting powder, he was of the notable sixteenth century alchemists.

Edward Kelly, another noble of sixteenth century appeared to have produced some Red and White elixirs. Elias Ashmole wrote at the end of his 'Theatrum Chemicum Britannicum' on Sir Edward Kelly's work which says: "*It is generally reported that Doctor Dee and Sir Edward Kelly were so strangely fortunate as to find a very large quantity of the Elixir in some part of the ruins of Glastonbury Abbey, which was so incredibly rich in virtue (being one in 272,330), that they lost much in making projection by way of trial before they finally found out the true height of the medicine.*"

In seventeenth century, Thomas Vaughan, wrote dozens of influential treatises on alchemy.

From England, there is also the story of a transmutation performed before King Gustavus Adolphus in 1620, the gold of which was coined into medals, bearing the king's effigy with the reverse Mercury and Venus; and of another at Berlin before the King of Prussia.

Modern Alchemy

Today the process of changing one fundamental substance into another is called Nuclear Physics. In the generation of Enriched nuclear fuels one basic substance will "miraculously" change into another. In a nuclear reactor, uranium is transmuted into plutonium, cesium, strontium, barium, iodine, krypton and xenon, to name but a few elements. These often decay to other stable elements through various radioactive processes. Such nuclear reactions are used to produce americium-241 for use in household smoke detectors, technetium-99 for use as a radioactive tracer in health care, and in production of plutonium-239- the isotope of plutonium used in nuclear weapons. In 1980, Glenn Seaborg was successful in transmuting minute quantities lead to gold, possibly via bismuth. In 1972, Russian scientists found that the lead shielding of an experimental nuclear reactor near Lake Baikal in Siberia had unexpectedly turned into gold! A possible route to gold would be from mercury. If mercury or its various naturally occurring isotopes could be made to capture neutrons, the resulting nuclear decay chains would eventually yield gold-197, the most common naturally occurring gold isotope, and perfectly stable. However the high cost of the transmutation is not economically viable.

Alchemy, though it largely passed from popularity, continued on. There have been experiments, even into the 20th century, that attempted transmutation, notably using nuclear power and particle acceleration. Pharmacology, while not necessarily admitting to any relationship with alchemy, has as its mission to find the "magic" drugs to help prolong life and heal sickness in much the same way alchemy operated 100s of years ago.

3

Principles of Spagyrics

"Alchemy is the gentle acceleration of growth through the use of the fire of nature." — *Paracelsus"*

In the ancient concept, what Nature delivered in the form specified in evolutionary process of living and non-living entities after complex processing and governed by the laws of interaction of a set of fundamental principles (Mercury, Sulphur and Salt) through the primordial elements that express the universal root (Water, Air, Fire, Earth).

This is a not insignificant aspect because it is the pivot around which Spagyric the Doctrine of the past has developed all the concepts related to the search of symptoms and their care through the appropriate remedy. Not only that, but as we previously seen, the transition from a cosmological-mythical view to a Systematic-experimental approach only takes place after a partial transformation of interior concepts gained on the basis of 'technical experience.

Established with the 'intent to develop medicines geared to the physical nature of the three Kingdoms (mineral and metal in particular) it becomes progressively Discipline Search in order to find a connection between the universal macrocosmic size and Human microcosm in all its reality signified. The Spagyria comes first as Spagyric Art with the aim of extracting from the mixed, or from complex bodies offered by Nature, under a 'unique form marked by three of' traditional principles of Alchemy Aristotelian matrix, the Quintessence or active spiritual substance, formed by the Spirit and from 'Soul, developed by dense and terrestrial matters fixed by Salt and animated by Spiritus mundi or vital fluid.

This conception that we will resume for a 'more detailed analysis in the study the process of genesis and evolution of the concept of Spagyric principles, see the Quintessences and other dynamized substances like regenerating the human body through communication of a surplus of vital energy and health. Through this process, therefore, the Spagyrist and the patient are both exposed to a phenomenon of controlled assimilation of the intrinsic virtues of the active ingredient extracted and reworked: the first because objectively extrinsic, first, act of placing itself in the preparation of the remedy tuning fork with the energetic reality of the transformation, the second because it assumes the 'object of the transformation that transforms in him the virtues acquired.

Now, experimentation has shown us that there are really principles; phytochemicals and active minerals with the 'body', but it would be rash to push too far this design and see something magical and miraculous. Our intention is to return Spagyrics according to the canons of a Science, but we do not want to make it a reality gold and detached from the global dimension of being, as it is not actually.

An important element is thus enclosed in the right placement of appropriate language. The laws of 'systematic analogy may come to us in aid.

First, there is a very strong link between the psychic dimension and size physiological; are not "bodies" separate or distinct, is all 'one', one reality constituted three types of interactions that we could easily assimilate to the Three Principles or Essential Tradition of Paracelsus. Such interactions are:

Inside the body, in which the organs occupy a particular geometry and are arranged according to a specific architecture (the fixed nature of sulfur).

Outside the body, instead of the external influences, the 'area' geometric that occupies the body and through which the pathogens are transmitted (The volatile nature, unstable and mercurial).

In psychological point of view, universe, the human mind, home of' life energy, the principle unifying par excellence, the one that regulates every function is through 'conscious processing through the 'unconscious in its broadest sense (the Salt, the fundamental balance principle that partakes of both previous).

In this fundamental perspective, just one even minimum level imbalance psychic to determine the pathological state.

By this we do not ever say that every disease originates the state of disruption in the mind channels, but we all know that the spirit endowed with reason, to quote Hahnemann, he lives a living organism animated by a 'Vital energy immaterial and we happily call dynamic of Existing'. And the rupture of 'balance of' vital energy which is the basis of the disease and who manifested through the disruption of the functions and sensations of the body.

Alchemy is one of the most ancient sciences, religions, and systems of medicine in the world. It is in essence the art of transformation. Most people perceive alchemy as "turning lead into gold," and while this is a minor aspect of the alchemical arts, it is something much deeper. It is not so much about making gold for monetary gain, but more about transmuting the base metal of our ego into the gold of our spirit. It is a systematic spirituality that brings one into harmony with the elements, the planets, and the source of creation.

There are three main branches of alchemy: the traditional western esoteric system, Ayurveda, and Taoist Chinese medicine. Each branch extends deep into the mysteries of nature and healing. But they are all branches reaching out of the same trunk with its roots deep in nature.

Alchemy provides an energetic cosmology, or map of the universe in which all things can be understood. This natural philosophy shows the energetic architecture from which all things are composed of. By understanding cosmology, we understand where we come from and where we are going- and the transformative process of where we are.

Spagyrics is the practical application of the cosmology of alchemy. One is theory, the other is practice. Spagyrics is a process of creating philosophical medicines that are made in harmony with the nature of the substance being worked with- mainly minerals, metals and plants. The word spagyrics comes from two Greek words "Spao" meaning to separate, and "gyro" meaning to combine. Thus, a certain natural substance is separated into its principle components, exhalted or concentrated, and recombined into a higher state of being. A true spagyricist not only purifies and evolves a piece of matter, but is purifying and evolving themselves with it. This is what makes alchemy a true spiritual system, that everything done in the external is also done in the internal and thus the medicine in embodied. This is the method in which all of the Organic Unity products are prepared.

The 'traditional Spagyrical concept inherited from 'conceptual framework of' Traditional alchemy address exoteric, the principle that the material world is a primordial substance or primitive but has a potential existence only as long as does not receive the 'footprint of a form, is the basic starting point for the' elaborating the concept of element and principle at the Ancients. It is good that you know that Aristotle considered the 'appearance formal aspect of reality not as Structural able to hit the five senses and give us back a feeling of a verifiable physical presence that causes rupture in the continuity of space (the "outer form", for instance); the form is for the greek philosopher all that gives to a body its specific qualities.

In its simplest manifestation, the form had originated from Four elements constituent, Fire, Air, Earth and Water, among them differentiated by quality.

The four attributes in original are: the fluidity or humidity, the dryness, the heat and the cold. However, Heating, Cooling, Wet and Dry, being opposed to each other can not be coupled; there are so only possible combinations:

Hot - Dry

Heat - Fluid - Wet

Cold - Fluid - Wet

Cold - Dry

In each element of an attribute predominates over the other: in the Dry Land, in 'Water its Moist, in Air Fluidity, the Fire Heat'. None of the four elements is immutable. mutual mutation could take place through the 'common attribute; so the Fire can become air by means of heat, the Air by means of fluidity can becoming water, etc.

Two elements may give rise to a third off each of its own quality attribute, provided that the operation does not produce two identical attributes or antonyms. In all these changes is not the matter primigenial to undergo the transformation, but the reality formal, which assumes a constant process of adaptation to different interactive conditions between himself and the size gained. Aristotle deduces from this process that every substance bears in itself, as a structural composition and structured, each Element defined and that the difference between the same substances derived from the diversity of Elements of proportional content.

The example of green wood burning is the most trivial form of water droplets to cut end of the branch because the wood contains water; are released smoke and vapors because it contained Air, combustion takes place because it contains fire, you get the ashes because the wood contains Earth. From this assumption, the classification of substances made by Aristotle it responds to the figure of the metaphysical rather than the quality experimental data based on the phenomena of chemical reactivity or, for the pure elements, on the given the atomic number as according to the fundamental concept of Principle.

The three fundamental principles were designed from data of Unit Matter : matter is as Essential primary and Semenza structures differentiated and for that reason can have a formal character infinity through mutual interaction of the constituent elements.

According to M. S Endivogius (1566-1646):

'the Tria Prima constituents, in their balance, the formal-structural data the mineral, vegetable and animal matter are spiritual entities already contained in power in the primordial material forming.

Matter, therefore, it is initially differentiate in Sulfur and Mercury, the non halogen element and the metal sublimable known to us, but two reality whose constitution takes part of the virtues of the Fire and dell 'Acqua, balanced by the quality Earthy and from the Air, which in different proportions would form the overall texture the differentiated body. These bodies are not chemical entities but can be isolated and exalted by the Art because content in the form settled all internal matter entitatively organized.'

The *Tria First*, the three principles, are in turn essential points of reference for the understanding of the structural data. They play an important role especially in the scientific review of Spagyria, the work of many of the seventeenth and nineteenth century researchers, as well as contemporary Spagyrists of French and US area involved particularly in understanding these data, as they will be stripped of many of their metaphysical categories of characteristics to take more concrete and adaptability. But for Paracelsus, the *Tria Prima* are still spiritual substances and not products concrete dell 'chemical analysis, but can be separated from the parent body if properly treated. They give to the material structure and functions, and are qualitatively different in the various bodies with regard to the diversity of substances which belong, though not negligible factor against what was stated by the Alchemy Traditional around the universal identity of structuring principles. So the specific features of the various bodies are in close relation with the constitution and defined structure of the same contents Principles, an element which seems open a matter of contradiction in Paracelsus' Doctrine and that in any case will not be never entirely clear in the dell 'German Author works. An important fact is that the extension of the Doctrine *Tria first* to allow the human microcosm approach Therapeutic Spagyrico, surpassing chemical and inorganic sense the conception umoralistica the originating tradition by Galen.

The spagyric medication obtained from the plant or mineral kingdom were therefore specifications obtained from the extraction and reprocessing of Tria Prima Body starting, identified on the basis of the Theory of Signatures, and therefore perfectly adaptable to the global organic structure of Man.

The decisive passage to a new conception of the Tria Prima Paracelsians happens, not without difficulty, taking up the J B van Helmont (1579-1644) theory and adapting it to 'modern experimental field, Alkemi shall develop a system epistemological and technical to open the perspectives d 'investigative and objective identification to a scientific definition of the principles in question. This moment of rupture takes place in a 'time when the Spagyria el' Alchemy They are progressively re-evaluated from a technical point of view to the work of the various organizations, the US first and foremost, that define a new method d 'approach. The chemist Belgian, animated by a particular desire for the definition specific areas, makes her the 'axiom of R. Boyle:

> *"The book of nature is a big and beautiful 'tapestry that we can not see it all in once, but we must be content to await the discovery of her beauty and its symmetry gradually."*

The fact that he chose this way of thinking and acting indicates right away and so effectively the versatility of his mind and the experimental tenacity with which he approached the Spagyric problems. His experimental philosophy, which is the general conception of Alchemical universe, whose symmetry is revealed through a patient verification work, you are moving in three directions.

The certainty of finding natural reason of symmetry and of harmony of interactions cosmic advocated by the ancients. The belief that one thorough study of organized matter, is theoretical and practical-experimental, can be the unique key for the solution of the problem.

The possibility of producing, through a review and an adaptation epistemological spagyrical discipline with other Sciences, a summary full and susceptible to continuous progress can contribute to wellbeing of humanity.

The three philosophical principles of alchemy are considered the working units of this system. It is the holy trinity of the universe. They are primary organic functions that exist within all of manifest creation- be it material or non-material. Understanding these principles assist in understanding the underlying patterns behind all things. Our minds are under their influence, as well as our physical bodies and emotional states. The planets, the plants, the minerals, the animals,spirits and non-physical beings are composed of the principles. The fact that all of existence contains these primary organic functions is what makes them universal.

All things contain various concentrations of each of the principles. While there are many energetic factors going into all manifestations (elements, planets, astrological archetypes, etc.), the three principles are the easiest to recognize as they are simple, non-specific, and observable. They are non-specific in the sense that there are only three to observe, and determine which is the most prominent, as compared to a planetary perspective where there are 7 (or 10) to decipher.

Majority of traditional cultures, cosmologies, and systems of medicines contain some form of the three principles. In the Ayurvedic tradition it is vata, pitta, and kapha. In astrology, it is mutable, cardinal, and fixed. In the western alchemical tradition, it is mercury, sulfur, and salt. In molecular science it is the proton, neutron, and electron. These are all the exact same things, just seen though different cultural perspectives and expressed in different languages.

When one begins to see and experience these three principles, the entire world begins to transform. Seeing the interrelatedness of all things unfolds, and patterns begin to emerge from the previously chaotic and random sequences of events and experiences. A certain magic is reinstated onto the world. The three principles are a universal language that nature speaks to us and relays qualitative information. We are able to tap into a higher order of the way things truly are.

When studying the three universal principles from the western alchemical tradition, it is important to remember that what is being spoken of is not chemical mercury, sulfur, and salt, but philosophical mercury, sulfur and salt. While these principles have their reflections in the chemicals they are named after, they have much broader application than mere chemistry. They are most useful in the study of botanical anatomy, that is, the inherent qualities and characteristics of a plant, as well as our own anatomy.

Another way to perceive these principles is through their elemental mothers. Each principle is a harmony of two elements (Earth, Air, Fire, Water). By understanding their elemental parents, their qualities of their being is able to be understood on a deeper level.

To get the most holistic understanding of the three universal principles, it is helpful to study their nature from the different systems that use them. In the Organic Unity paradigm, we work mostly with the western alchemical tradition, Ayurveda, and Astrology. Each system allows insights into the principles that the others may fail to notice and thus broadens the perspective.

Sulfur

Sulfur is a harmony of the Air and Fire elements. In that way, it is moveable, penetrating, hot, and diffusive. Within the human body, the Sulfur principle is reflected as our soul. The soul under this definition is our own unique expression of the life force. It is our individuality, our true essential nature, our essence. It is the flame of our awareness. The correlation with Air is that our soul is not limited to our body, it has the ability to leave the body through astral projection, dream travel, and visionary journeying.

This can be better understood when looking at the Sulfur principle within plants, which is reflected in its volatile (essential) oils. The essential oil of a plant is a reflection of its essence. It is that plant's unique flavor. When one smells an essential oil of Rheum palmatum for example, you are connecting with that plant's unique identity; there is no other smell on the face of the planet that smells like it. It is the dynamic expression of the life force within that particular plant. Like Fire and Air, the essential oils of a plant volatilize very easily (they disperse through the air) and they are often very heating and intense.

Chemical Sulfur, as most people know, smells very strong and tends to permeate the surrounding space and penetrate sharply. It ignites very easily, and puts our a very hot, bright flame.

Mercury

The Mercury principle is composed of the Water and Air elements, and as such, is a mediator between the volatile or etheric elements, and the fixed elements. In traditional Greek mythology, Mercury was the messenger of the gods, and was in constant movement between the above and the below. Within the human body, Mercury is the spirit, or the animating life force. Whereas Sulfur is the soul, or the consciousness of the individual, Mercury is the life force that move through the soul and gives it life. As the mediator, it is the vehicle that brings the soul down into the physical world.

Within the botanical kingdom, Mercury is reflected in the alcohol and water soluble constituents of the plant, called secondary metabolites in pharmacognosy. If one takes any plant on the face of the planet and ferment it, which in alchemy is considered a death (it putrefies or rots), one yields ethyl alcohol, but puts a plant through a sort of death experience, and what is released is alcohol, which is the same in every plant. The spirit is released. This is why alcohol is commonly called spirits. So the spirit of the plant is the alcohol and water components of the plant. This is highly mercurial in nature because alcohol tends to extract more volatile (Air) constituents (resins, essential oils) and water tends to extract more fixed (Water) constituents (polysaccharides, glycosides, alkaloids). Thus, the spirit, or Mercury of a plant brings together or harmonizes the two sides of the spectrum of botanical constituents.

Chemical Mercury is an interesting substance. It is the only liquid metal and is highly moveable, changeable, and volatile- turns to vapor (Air) very quickly. It is somehow solid, yet liquid at the same time, and also moves into a gas.

Salt

So we have the soul (Sulfur) and the spirit (Mercury), and finally we come to salt- the crystallization, the manifestation, the vehicle through which the more subtle principles work through. Each principle progressed through various levels of density, with salt being the most dense. It is composed of the Water and Earth elements.

Salt in the human is reflected as the physical body, and is thus infinitely complex. Millions of chemical reactions occurring each second, most of which we know nothing about. The human body is one of the most beautiful mysteries we may ever come to know, a microcosm of the universe. It is the anchor for our soul and spirit, the temple in which they reside.

In botanical kingdom, the Salt principle is reflected in the mineral matrix of the plant. These are obtained through certain extraction methods using the Fire and Water elements to crystallize pure mineral salts. As with the human, these minerals are the vehicle through which the Sulfur (essential oil) and the Mercury (alcohol/water solubles) principles work through.

As far as botanical extracts go, it is these three principles that are primarily worked with their preparation. Each principle of a plant is separated and purified, and then the three are reunited. This is the principle behind spagyrics- to separate and recombine.

Most conventional herbal tinctures contain only the Mercury and Sulfur components of a plant. They macerate the herb in an alcohol and water menstruum for a period of time, filter the liquid material out and compost or throw away the solid plant material. Thus, majority of tinctures are missing 1/3 of a plant's constituents, the mineral body through which the other constituents work through. It is disembodied medicine.

This is not to say that herbal tinctures do not work, they absolutely work and have provided an amazing service to the world by providing a natural means to palliate symptoms and heal their bodies. But in a sense, they are not able to work as well on our physical bodies as they could because they themselves are missing their physical bodies. The addition of the Salt principle to a tincture greatly enhances its effectiveness and potency and thus lower doses are often needed.

> *"The term spagyric is often used as a synonym for alchemy. More accurately, it has also come to mean the practical application of alchemy to the creation of medicinal remedies. According to alchemy the Cosmos, which encompasses all of existence, was created by the Divine and has 3 main spheres of existence: spirit – soul – body.*
>
> *Essentially, the perfect spirit is purely objective and timeless. Light is a metaphor for the perfect spirit. Interestingly, even physics recognizes light as a timeless phenomenon that never changes in the course of time. Alchemy regards the soul and physical matter as condensed light. Thus spirit causes matter: spirit › soul › body. According to the theory of relativity, energy (light) is changeable into matter (material) and vice versa. For instance;*
>
> *– The sun is losing 4.2 million tons of matter per second through processes of nuclear fusions, which frees energy.*
>
> *"All matter originates and exists only by virtue of vibration." - Max Planck (Nobel Prize winner and the father of Quantum Physics).*

– By means of particle accelerators, particles with almost the speed of light can be fired and be brought to collision. This way the kinetic energy can be released into new and measurable parts.

"natural science of the present, which is still spiritually alienated despite quantum mechanics and the theory of relativity." - Alexander von Bernus

In the perfect cosmos, matter (soul and body) is completely spiritualized. In this manner, totally spiritualized matter transmits the perfect light to the outside (soul > body). In spagyric remedies, water and alcohol have this transmitting characteristic! This transmuting of spirit into matter through specific processes is what Spagyric Medicine is based on.

Each life rhythm – as for example the rhythms of day and night, the rhythm of the seasons, the rhythm of the years, the rhythm of life, rhythms of the heart and the breath, etc. – has two phases: In the rhythm of mercurial expansion and saline phase of densification, the nature of things is changed into the direction of predestined perfection and complete health.

In the expansion phase (which is derived through distillation of medicinal plants) the activating mercurius operates. It dissolves matter (soul and body), thus dissolving the materialized forms of life. This way spirit is separated from matter (Spa from Greek = separate). The energy freed from matter can enter the perfect spiritual light (the universal ether) and can become potentiated.

In the densification phase (which is brought about through the process of maceration) the retarding Sal operates. It concentrates matter (soul, body) and thereby connects the previously heightened form of spirit with matter (gyrik from Greek = connect). This way the spirit forms of life reach matter (soul and body).

In the rhythm of mercurial expansion and saline phase of densification, the nature of things is changed into the direction of predestined perfection and complete health."

(*Spagyric and the Cosmos Universe* - Christoph Proeller, Paracelsus-Magazine, Büelstrasse, Hergiswil)

Human being, as a living, thinking, feeling, vibrating being, are much more than a collection of interlinked chemical processes. Every thought, emotion, vibration or action leads to a series of chemical changes in the body. All ailments are a result of disharmony in the life force. Spagyrics restores this imbalance in the life force, bringing mind, body and soul into harmony. Treating an ailment on a molecular level alone, seldom has a lasting effect as the untreated social, emotional, mental, spiritual and energetic patterns cause the ailment to manifest once again on a physical plane. Spagyrics balance the energetic and the physiological manifestation of the five elements; and micronutrients to coordinate cellular nutrition.

4

The Simila of Alchemy

The theory that like can be treated with like can be traced back as far Hippocrates (468-377 BC),"Many before Hahnemann, from Hippocrates down, had glimpses of the law [of similars], and some had tried to make use of it therapeutically;" - Close [1924, p. 215]. "Paracelsus was also a firm believer in the doctrine of signatures, and in illustration of it explained every single part of St. John's Wort (Hypericum perforatum) in terms of this belief "the holes in the leaves mean that this herb helps all inner and outer orifices of the skin, the blooms rot in the form of blood, a sign that it is good for wounds and should be used where flesh has to be treated." [Griggs, 1981]

"Though Hahnemann may not have intended to carry into his new system any of the ideas of alchemy, there seems little doubt that several of its techniques did get carried in, intentionally or otherwise. Indeed, he seems to have taken many of the techniques of alchemy, dumped the theories and used the techniques to prepare his new remedies, chosen on the basis of the law of similars." [Morrell, 1999]

The principles underlying homeopathy can be traced to roots dating back even further than those of immunology. Mankind has always wondered how to identify remedies capable of curing diseases. In the pre-scientific era, empiricism based on chance observations, and trial and error, was probably the most widely used approach, accompanied by various forms of oral or written tradition. In many other cases, the sick relied (and still do among some primitive people) on the intuition of individuals judged to be particularly endowed with divine or natural powers: healers, shamans, witch-doctors and so on. However, there was also another line of thought that, often in a marginal manner, has accompanied various medical cultures in different epochs: the identification of particular 'resemblances' between remedies and the diseases they were thought to be able to cure. The first examples of treating 'like with like' can be found in the papyrus of Ebers (1500 BC): ear diseases treated with ear extracts, headache with fish heads, blindness with the eyes of a pig.

Attempting to treat a disease by administering the agent capable of causing it or transmitting it is one of the most general acquisitions of empirical medicine. Numerous primitive medicines used to cure the effects of snake venoms by repeatedly inoculating them or materials extracted from the snake venom. In the Far East the Chinese practiced a form of preventive smallpox vaccination both by wearing the clothes worn by a smallpox victim in the full suppuration phase of the disease and by inhaling dried smallpox pustules after storing them for 1 year. Pliny claimed that the saliva of a rabid dog can afford protection against rabies. Dioskurides of Anazarbo recommended that hydrophobia sufferers eat the liver of the dog that bit them. Aetius of Antioch recommended eating the meat of the viper that had just bitten you. In the seventeenth century the Irishman Robert Fludd cured the victims of consumption with dilutions of their own sputum after suitable preparation.

Equally primitive and often elaborate applications of the same principle could be found in many pharmacopoeias until the last century. The reasoning is sometimes elementary: swallow human stones in cases of calculosis but, also here, the connection is obscure in the light of current knowledge. It is well known that King Mithridates VI (132-163 BC) is said to have taken small quantities of poisons and toxins to protect himself against the repeated attempts made to poison him. Native Americans wear a headdress of eagle feathers partly to underline their prowess as hunters and partly for decorative purposes, but the custom is also based on a belief that the sight, speed, courage and other desirable characteristics of the eagle can be magically acquired. The magical transfer of the courage of a killed enemy to the victor by means of the ingestion of organs (the heart) also explains some aspects of cannibalism.

The 'Simile' of Hippocrates

By means of highly acute observations made without sophisticated instruments but still valid today, the school of Hippocrates understood that many of the phenomena of a disease are attempts at cure and suggested imitating them: this is the Hippocratic 'simile'. The most frequently cited assertions are:

The pains (complaints) will be removed by means of their opposite, each according to its own characteristics. Thus, heat corresponds to a hot constitution that has been made ill by the cold, and so on for the others. Another way of removing pain is the following: a disease develops by means of its like and is cured by means of the use of its like. Thus, what causes urinary tenesmus in health cures it in disease. Cough is caused and cured by means of the same agent, as in the case of urinary tenesmus. Another method: the fever causing the development of inflammation will be caused and cured by the same agent. At other times, it will be cured by the opposite of its cause [Littre's *Oeuvres Completes d'Hippocrates*, VI, 334, Paris, 1839].

It is particularly worth mentioning that Hippocrates did not adopt a dogmatic or ideological position, but saw both approaches ('similarity' and 'opposition') as potentially useful. Prognostic interest, a great capacity for controlled observation, the rejection of fanciful tendencies and other characteristics unmistakably distinguish this from magic.

Without going into the whole of Hippocratic medicine, it must be said that his doctrine is permeated by the concept of natural healing. Nature ('physis') is the healer of disease. 'Physis' is an expression of life, not a special energy; it is unconscious or similar to instinct; it prevails over physiological and mechanical processes; it combats disease; it is frequently incomplete and must be assisted by a doctor. It is likely that no thought has had a more profound effect on medicine than Hippocrates observation that the manifestations of disease consist of two groups of events: the first being the direct effects of the damage, the second the reaction of repair. The corollary to this is that the direct effects must be removed whenever possible, but the reparative reaction must be promoted in order to imitate nature. Hippocrates considered many pathophysiological phenomena as being fundamentally 'defensive': fever, skin eruptions and others. In line with this pathophysiological conception, physicians must make a distinction between useful and harmful symptoms by stimulating the former and blocking the latter. Using typical Greek conciseness, Hippocrates formulated what can legitimately be considered one of the fundamental rules of therapy: nature is the primary physician and the first duty of medicine is 'to do no harm'.

The 'Simile' of Paracelsus

One further representative of this line of thought was P.T. von Hohenheim, also known as Paracelsus. His works, which were first published in Basel in an almost complete version of 11 volumes between 1589 and 1591, contain a mixture of genial intuitions and ingenuities; profound clinical observations and strange affirmations concerning the influence of celestial bodies; new pharmacological observations and convinced assertions as to the truth of alchemical and magical concepts. Among other things, Paracelsus proposed the 'doctrine of signatures' ('signa naturae') according to which the therapeutic properties of different remedies were 'similar' to and could be deduced from the external appearance of plants and minerals: red remedies for blood diseases, sharply pointed leaves for the pain caused by stab wounds, iris-colored Eufrasia for eye diseases, topaz against jaundice (because both are yellow) and so on. In this way, 'magical similarity' was re-exhumed in an empirical and intuitive manner without any scientific understanding or experimental proof.

However, not all of the work of Paracelsus was 'magical': he had many important intuitions and made a number of empirical observations that were to form the basis for a large number of medical applications in subsequent centuries. For a long time, the following citation was considered one of the most significant anticipations of the 'simile' as seen by homeopathy: 'What causes jaundice also cures jaundice'. That is, the good and the bad lie in the same thing: the bad causes jaundice but, if you separate the good, it becomes an efficacious remedy against jaundice. Since the drugs that cure paralysis must come from the substances that cause it. This is the way to understand the curative powers of minerals. What may be harmful in our hands can be transformed into a medicine' [Paracelsus, Miners Diseases, IX, 481]. There is also a certain harmony with the concepts concerning drug doses that were subsequently adopted by homeopaths, since according to Paracelsus medicines must be administered not on the basis of their weight, but according to criteria that go beyond simple weight.

In the post-Paracelsian period, the 'simile' was often mentioned, but usually in reference to magical practices. Typical authors are Porta, who attempted to apply the doctrine of signatures to the whole botanic world (examples include the use of hairy plants for scalps, beautiful plants to improve personal appearance, 'happy' plants, 'sad' plants, etc.), and Schroder who presented related ideas, such as the fact that the leaves of Hepatica triloba resemble the liver. One true predecessor of Hahnemann was Stoerck (1731-1803), who in the 1760s published a series of works on the treatment of diseases with poisons according to the principle of similars. This author made a highly significant statement: 'If stramonium causes illness in someone who is sound in mind by inducing mental confusion, why should we not try to establish whether it can give mental health to someone who is confused or whose senses are altered by disease? If it cures someone affected by spasms, why should we not investigate whether it causes the spasms?'

Paracelsus also extended his belief on the doctrine of the Signature. This is named as the Paracelsian simile. His examples are vast. The plant Cyclamen used for ear diseases as the leaf looks like human ear. The yellow remedies used for jaundice due to their resemblance in colour. Hahnemann himself used to believe this as a source of materia medica and sited a huge number of examples in his literature.

The work of Paracelsus, in many paragraphs opposed the contraria principle. Some of them read like the following:

"It is true that he, who will employ cold for the heat, Moister for dryness, does not, understood the nature of the disease."

"What makes jaundice that also cures jaundice. The medicine that shall cure paralysis must produce from that causes it".

"When Antimony is ingested it produces cough, great hardness of stool, so it will cure the similar condition".

"Alkali cures oppression of breathing - so it will cure the similar condition". About similia he states,

"What makes jaundice also heals Jaundice. This is good and bad are in the same thing; out of the bad comes jaundice; but if the good separates, then it is the Arcanum (remedy) against jaundice – because the drugs which would heal paralysis must come out of the same which causes it – so that Arcane (healing power) of minerals become understood, so that Gold as a remedy for all diseases of those who seek after it. So also saturnus has its Arcanum which, goes out of lead – what may be damaging in our hands will also be changed through our hands into a drug".

Hahnemann wrote totally different, however is the result when two similar diseases meet together in the organism, that is to say, when to the diseases already present a stronger similar is added. We see how a cure can be affected by the operations of nature, and we get a lesion as to how man ought to cure (*Organon of medicine*, 5th and 6th Edn. Economic Homoeo Publishers, Kolkata, 2004, p. 278, also Aph. 38 of the 4th Edition, pp. 116–117). "A weaker dynamic affection is permanently extinguished in the living organism by a stronger one, if the latter (whilst differing in kind) is very similar to the former in its manifestations" (*Organon of Medicine*, Hahnemann, 5th and 6th Edn, Translation By R. E. Dudgeon and William Boericke, B. Jain, New Delhi, 1996). Hahnemann substantiated numbers of examples in footnote 2 of the same section and the examples regarding diseases came in aphorism 46 (*History of Homoeopathy*, Linn J. Boyd, Ibid, p. 218). Hahnemann in Medicine of Experience mentioned this maxim in a different manner, say; it is only by this property of producing in the healthy body a series of specific morbid symptoms, that medicines can cure diseases, that is to say, remove and extinguish the morbid irritation by a suitable counter-irritant (*The Medicine of Experience*, Lesser writings, Hahnemann, Ibid, page- 451).

5

Difference Between Homoeopathy and Spagyric Homoeopathy

Spagyrics or Plant Alchemy as the medicine has been created by Paracelsus more than 500 years ago, and Homeopathy has been developed by Hahnemann 200 years ago.

Homoeopathic mother tincture is made from plant or other natural source. All plants go through the process of maceration for making the liquid homoeopathic mother tinctures. After being chopped the fresh plants pieces are placed into a hermetically lockable glass-encased grinder together with alcohol. Pure alcohol is used because it is the most effective solvent for extracting the plant's bio-active constituents and delivering them into the bloodstream and across the cell membrane quickly. Many of the plant's constituents are poorly soluble in water, such as resins, essential oils and most alkaloids.

Then the solution or mixture is placed in a dark container or space so that the chemical constituents of the plant are not destroyed. The soaking process can take weeks or even months depending on the substance.

Spagyric essences are made from plants by a unique process, which neutralise their toxic components, but preserves their healing potential. It is concentrated essence, sometimes light coloured with the flavour and smells. So the difference between Spagyric and homeopathy is even apparent to our senses, a homeopathic remedy being hardly differentiable by color, smell or taste from a water-alcohol solution.

Spagyrics means separate and recombine, and can be used to make herbal extracts of great power and energetic force.

Homeopathic mother tinctures are diluted usually in alcohol, then using successive dilutions and succussions of this "mother tincture" potentised dilutions are created with a static or frozen vibrational signature of the original material used, but with none of its physical characteristics.

This misperception occurs more and more often as large European pharmaceutical companies realize the profitability of taking labour-intensive Spagyric mother solutions and stretching them into sometimes thousands of gallons of sellable homeopathic product. The facilitation of physical and spiritual healing is there is no reason to potentise Spaygyric essence, as through the circulation process it gets potentised and becomes full of healing potential and the vital strength of the plant.

Plant Alchemy or Spagyrics represents a form of homeopathy in which both vital healing energy and active substances are extracted from medicinal plants, creating powerful mother tinctures that can be further potentized by the circulation process. Derived from the Greek words spao (separate) and ageiro (unite), spagyric remedies were originally created by fermenting parts of wild herbs. This process produced concentrated aromatic solutions that were extracted and separated from the bulk plant matter. After fermentation was completed, the plant material was distilled in a special device, and the remainder dried and burned. The ashes were extracted and purified via distillation, then recombined with the concentrated solution. As a result, the finished spagyric essence contained the mineral constituent parts of the plant. Paracelsus pointed out that the vital energy of an herb is more important than the plant material itself. Spagyric remedies undergo six key steps: separation, purification, distillation, incineration, re-unification and circulation.

Homoeopathic Mother Tinctures and Spagyric Tinctures have some key differences which could be checked by observing rule of three, Aroma, Taste and Color or physical appearance. Homoeopathic mother tinctures are either straw or tea liquor colored with no specific taste or aroma of the concerned plant, whereas, Spagyric Tinctures bear the specific aroma of the plant, tastes sweet, besides light colored or colorless. Spagyric essences, through the circulation process gets potentised, alike Homeopathy potentisation is not required. Spagyrics means plant alchemy, wherein no minerals or chemicals are processed, it is covered in another segment of Alchemy which is known as Metal or Mineral Alchemy.

Spagyric forms a bridge between classical homoeopathy and modern plants science. Although these are two seperate sciences.

The energy of the Cosmos is captured in nature. Spagyric uses these forces of nature to eliminate the blockades, deficits and other pathogenic factors that cause disease

The use of Spagyric works on the spiritual, mental and physical level. The choice of the elements their relationship and degree of dosage determines what happens.

Spagyric extracts hit a diseased person like a cosmic thunderbolt of healing energy. Spagyrics "opens" the plant and liberates medicine powers not available in the ordinary extract. These medicine powers have nothing to do with the pharmacologically active constituents modern science seeks to standardize.

Both spagyric and ordinary extraction methods macerate (soak) the herb in a menstrum (mixture) of water and grain alcohol between the new and full moon. Water dissolves the water-soluble nutrients; alcohol the alkaloids. The extract is then pressed out, leaving the plant fiber. With ordinary techniques, this fiber or marc is discarded, thus losing the many minerals, trace elements and nutrients, including glycosides, locked up in the cellulose matrix.

The spagyric method cremates the marc in an airtight, oxygen-free kiln at 1500 degrees Fahrenheit for a prolonged period of time (5 or 6 days). This calcination process produces a fine white, mineral rich alkaline ash that is then run (mixed) in a special kind of water, oscillated at a high frequency, pressed out, and allowed to dry into crystals.

Once this running in water process is completed a second time, the crystalline ash is recombined (reunited in the "chymical wedding") back into the original liquid extract, yielding an extremely high potency, fast-acting formula with the full synergy and aroma of the whole living herb and of the etheric cosmic forces that created it. Because of the distillation process Spagyric Homoeopathy retains the electrolyte properties of the plants and this is critical to the healing process.

Why are spagyric extracts infinitely more potent than ordinary ones? Because they release all the nutrients and minerals; because they work with the universal energies of the cosmos; and because they draw upon the spagyric practitioner's mindful intent and inspired heart.

Spagyric Homoeopathy is governed in Germany under section 39 of the Federal drug law. Zimpel, Krauss, Beyersdorff, Strathmeyer, Gluckselig and Bernus prescriptions are covered under this law.

Spagyric Homoeopathy is governed in United States of America vide Revision Service Official Compendium from July 1, 1992 pp. 34-35, December 1998 of the Homeopathic Pharmacopoeia of the United States (HPUS). Under this HPUS revision Zimpel, Krauss and Beyersdorff prescriptions are registered.

6

Botanical Consciousness in Spagyrics

As a natural and whole therapeutic system, Spagyric medicine offers a holistic solution to physical and psychological ailments. It treats the human being as a whole- body, soul and spirit - and in this respect, Spagyric has the same foundation as the oldest ways of healing mankind, namely Chinese, Tibetan and Ayurvedic medicines.

Plants are central to Spagyric medicine. Spagyric essences are made from plants, and a whole energetic medicine is based on the system, which has fundamental differences from herbalism. The spagyrist believes that a hidden therapeutic force resides within the plants. This force can be released and even increased by a complex process related to alchemy.

In the realm of working with the botanical kingdom, a great focus has been put on plant communication. This is a great step for humanity in that it brings us back to the realization that the natural world is latent with information and that we can in fact tap into that wisdom. But information really only grazes the surface, it does not penetrate to the depth of being. We don't really understand something until it has entered the realm of direct experience.

Every single aspect of a plant is communicating its intelligence to us in unique ways, myriads of forms. From its molecules, to its shape and structure, its environmental and habitat patterns, to its organ affinity and physical, mental, emotional and spiritual actions on the human organism. Everything about that plant is communication, and communication infers intelligence.

Through an understanding of a system of energetics, this intelligence is able to be mapped out, to be placed into some sort of workable pattern. Energetics is a system of natural language that effectively captures and embodies the essential nature of the botanical being and how it relates to the human being. This natural language is simple and understandable, because it is based off the observation of nature and the connections between its various forms. It connects seemingly disconnected things, thus revealing the unity of the natural world.

Establishing and building a relationship with a plant is very similar to doing the same with a human being: the first few interactions can be slow, steady and gradual. We will really hit it off with some plants, like we have known them for years others may take a little more time. Plants, like people, can be very outgoing, talkative and expressive, or they can be more quiet and reserved. Like any relationship, it has to be tended to and nourished; it is a discipline and spiritual practice.

Establishing a relationship with a plant is establishing a relationship with a particular aspect of our own being.

Ancient Alchemists were very careful in choosing the herbs for preparing their spagyric essences considering the color and planetary affiliations (*viz.* which herb is connected to which zodiac) of the herbs.

Biological pigments, also known simply as pigments or biochromes are substances produced by living organisms that have a color resulting from selective color absorption. Biological pigments include plant pigments and flower pigments. The primary function of pigments in plants is photosynthesis, which uses the green pigment chlorophyll along with several red and yellow pigments that help to capture as much light energy as possible.

Other functions of pigments in plants include attracting insects to flowers to encourage pollination.

Plant pigments include a variety of different kinds of molecule, including porphyrins, carotenoids, anthocyanins and betalains. All biological pigments selectively absorb certain wave-lengths of light while reflecting others.

Much research has been done on the effects of various light wave-lengths on plant growth. Different photosynthetic pigments within plants utilize different wavelengths and plants use those various wave-lengths to accomplish different growth and development processes.

Pigments are light absorbing molecules built into thylakoid membranes which absorb some wavelengths and reflect others, chloroplasts contain several kinds of pigments which absorb different wavelengths of light.

Pigment Color and Maximum Absoption

Violet: 400 - 420 nm

Indigo: 420 - 440 nm

Blue: 440 - 490 nm

Green: 490 - 570 nm

Yellow: 570 - 585 nm

Orange: 585 - 620 nm

Red: 620 - 780 nm

Chlorophyll A absorbs blue, violet and red light, it reflects green. Chlorophyll B absorbs blue and orange light, reflects yellow, green.

Ultraviolet Light (10nm-400nm)

Studies show that 385 nm UV light promotes the accumulation of phenolic compounds and enhances antioxidant activity of plant extracts.

Blue Light (430nm-450nm)

It enables cryptochromes and phototropins to mediate plant responses such as phototropic curvature, inhibition of elongation growth, chloroplast movement, stomatal opening and seedling growth regulation. It affects chlorophyll formation, photosynthesis processes, and through the cryptochrome and phytochrome system, raises the photomorphogenetic, response. These wave-lengths encourage vegetative growth through strong root growth and intense photosynthesis and are often used as supplemental light for seedlings and young plants during the vegetative stage of their growth cycle, especially when "stretching" must be reduced or eliminated.

Green Light (500nm-550nm)

It is sometimes used as a tool for eliciting specific plant responses such as stomatal control, phototropism, photomorphogenic growth and environmental signaling. When combined with blue, red and far-red wave-lengths, green light completes a comprehensive spectral treatment for understanding plant physiological activity.

Red light (640nm-680nm)

It affects phytochrome reversibility and is the most important for photosynthesis, flowering and fruiting regulation. These wavelengths encourage stem growth, flowering and fruit production, and chlorophyll production.

Far Red (730nm)

It has the strongest action on the far-red absorbing form of phytochrome, for plants requiring relatively low values of the phytochrome photoequilibrium to flower.

It seems strange that plants would harvest the lower energy red light instead of the higher energy green light, unless you consider that, like all life, plants first evolved in the ocean.

A recent research by NASA revealed that sea water quickly absorbs the red light, and it is only blue light which can penetrate to any depth. Since early plants and still most plant-life today, lived in the ocean, optimizing their pigments to absorb the reds and yellows that were present in ocean water was most effective

Spagyric medicine seeks to heal by employing the natural energy in plants, *viz*, the electrical impulses, nutrients, and energies inherent in all living plants.

Spagyric Essence reflect the unity of the three philosophical principles expressed through the crystallized mineral salts, alcohol and water soluble constituents, and the volatile oils of the plants or the Salt, Mercury, and Sulfur, respectively. Often requiring months of preparing, Spagyric Essences are prepared through various processes of distillation, fermentation, calcination, sublimation, and exhaltation, all done in accordance with the particular planetary archetype that corresponds to that plant. These are true whole plant extracts delivering the highest intelligence of the plants in concentrated form with nothing being isolated or neglected.

7

Micronutrients and Spagyrics

Over 30 micronutrients are essential for human health and for the proper growth and development of children. They are all vitamins and minerals available in foods. Micronutrient deficiencies are prevalent public health problems in many countries, especially developing countries.

The phrase "we are what we eat" is frequently used to signify that the composition of our bodies is dependent in large measure on what we have consumed. The many chemical elements in the human body occur mainly in the form of water, protein, fats, mineral salts and carbohydrates. Each human body is built up from food containing these five constituents, and vitamins as well.

Minerals have a number of functions in the body. Sodium, potassium and chlorine are present as salts in body fluids, where they have a physiological role in maintaining osmotic pressure. Minerals form part of the constitution of many tissues. For example, calcium and phosphorus in bones combine to give rigidity to the whole body. Minerals are present in body acids and alkalis; for example, chlorine occurs in hydrochloric acid in the stomach. They are also essential constituents of certain hormones, e.g. iodine in the thyroxine produced by the thyroid gland.

The principal minerals in the human body are calcium, phosphorus, potassium, sodium, chlorine, sulphur, copper, magnesium, manganese, iron, iodine, fluorine, zinc, cobalt and selenium. Phosphorus is so widely available in plants that a shortage of this element is unlikely in any diet. Potassium, sodium and chlorine are easily absorbed and are physiologically more important than phosphorus. Sulphur is consumed by humans mainly in the form of sulphur containing amino acids; thus sulphur deficiency, when it occurs, is linked with protein deficiency. Copper, manganese and magnesium deficiencies are not believed to be common. The minerals that are of most importance in human nutrition are thus calcium, iron, iodine, fluorine and zinc, and only these are discussed in some detail here. Some mineral elements are required in very tiny amounts in human diets but are still vital for metabolic purposes; these are termed "essential trace elements".

Calcium

Calcium is an essential mineral with a wide range of biological roles. Apart from being a major constituent of bones and teeth, calcium is crucial for muscle contraction, nerve conduction, the beating of the heart, blood coagulation, glandular secretion, the production of energy and the maintenance of immune function, among other things. Calcium is an alkaline-earth metal with atomic number 20 and an atomic mass of 40.08 daltons. Its atomic symbol is Ca.

The body of an average-sized adult contains about 1250 g of calcium. Over 99 percent of the calcium is in the bones and teeth, where it is combined with phosphorus as calcium phosphate, a hard substance that gives the body rigidity. However, although hard and rigid, the skeleton of the body is not the unchanging structure it appears to be. In fact, the bones are a cellular matrix, and the calcium is continuously taken up by the bones and given back to the body. The bones, therefore, serve as a reserve supply of this mineral.

Calcium is present in the serum of the blood in small but important quantities, usually about 10 mg per 100 ml of serum. There are also about 10 g of calcium in the extracellular fluids and soft tissues of the adult body.

In humans and other mammals, calcium and phosphorus together have an important role as major components of the skeleton. They are also important, however, in metabolic functions such as muscular function, nervous stimuli, enzymatic and hormonal activities and transport of oxygen.

Iron

Iron deficiency is a very common cause of ill health in all parts of the world. The average iron content in a healthy adult is only about 3 to 4 g, yet this relatively small quantity is vital.

Most of the iron in the body is present in the red blood cells, mainly as a component of haemoglobin. Much of the rest is present in myoglobin, a compound occurring mainly in muscles, and as storage iron or ferritin, mainly in the liver, spleen and bone marrow. Additional tiny quantities are found binding protein in the blood plasma and in respiratory enzymes.

The main, vital function of iron is in the transfer of oxygen at various sites in the body. Haemoglobin is the pigment in the erythrocytes that carries oxygen from the lungs to the tissues. Myoglobin in skeletal and heart muscle accepts the oxygen from the haemoglobin. Iron is also present in peroxidase, catalase and the cytochromes.

Iodine

The body of an average adult contains about 20 to 50 mg of iodine, much of it in the thyroid gland. Iodine is essential for the formation of thyroid hormones secreted by this gland.

In humans iodine functions as an essential component of the hormones of the thyroid gland, an endocrine gland situated in the lower neck. Thyroid hormones, of which the most important is thyroxine (T4), are important for regulating metabolism. In children they support normal growth and development, including mental development.

Fluorine

Fluorine is a mineral element found mainly in the teeth and skeleton. Traces of fluorine in the teeth help to protect them against decay. Some studies have suggested that fluoride may also help strengthen bone, particularly later in life, and may thus inhibit the development of osteoporosis.

Other Trace Elements

Numerous minerals are present in the human body. For most of the trace elements, besides those discussed above, there is no evidence that deficiency is responsible for major public health problems anywhere. Some of these minerals are very important in metabolism or as constituents of body tissues. Many of them have been studied, and their chemistry and biochemistry have been described. Experimental deficiencies have been produced in laboratory animals, but most human diets, even poor diets, do not appear to lead to important deficiencies. These minerals therefore are not of public health importance. Other trace elements are present in the body but do not have any known essential role. Some minerals, for example lead and mercury, are of great interest to health workers because excess intake has commonly resulted in toxic manifestations.

Cobalt, copper, magnesium, manganese and selenium deserve mention because of their important nutritional role, and lead and mercury because of their toxicity. These minerals are considered in detail in large comprehensive textbooks of nutrition.

Cobalt

Cobalt is of interest to nutritionists because it is an essential part of vitamin B_{12} (cyanocobalamin). When isolated as a crystalline substance, the vitamin was found to contain about 4 percent cobalt. However, cobalt deficiency does not play a part in the anaemia that results from vitamin B_{12} deficiency.

Silica

Silica is not present in the body in large amounts, yet is found in virtually every type of tissue in the body. Silica is used to keep bones, cartilage, tendons and artery walls healthy and may be beneficial in the treatment of allergies, heartburn and gum diseases, as well as assisting the immune system.

Molybdenum

Molybdenum is an essential trace mineral in animal and human nutrition. It is found in several tissues of the human body and is required for the activity of some enzymes that are involved in catabolism, including the catabolism of purines and the sulfur amino acids. Molybdenum is a transition metal with atomic number 42 and an atomic weight of 95.94 daltons. Its symbol is Mo. Compounds of molybdenum are among the scarcer constituents of the earth's crust. In fact, molybdenum is only about three times more abundant than gold. Organic forms of molybdenum are found in living matter, from bacteria to animals, including humans.

Chromium

Chromium is believed to be an essential trace mineral in human nutrition. Evidence suggests that it plays an important role in normal carbohydrate metabolism. In the 1950s it was found that chromium was necessary for the maintenance of normal glucose tolerance in rats; chromium deficient rats had impaired glucose tolerance. Subsequently, it was found that patients receiving long term total parenteral nutrition (TPN) without chromium developed glucose intolerance, weight loss and peripheral neuropathy. These symptoms were reversed when the patients were given intravenous chromium chloride.

Molybdenum

Molybdenum is an essential trace mineral in animal and human nutrition. It is found in several tissues of the human body and is required for the activity of some enzymes that are involved in catabolism, including the catabolism of purines and the sulfur amino acids. Molybdenum is a transition metal with atomic number 42 and an atomic weight of 95.94 daltons. Its symbol is Mo. Compounds of molybdenum are among the scarcer constituents of the earth's crust. In fact, molybdenum is only about three times more abundant than gold. Organic forms of molybdenum are found in living matter, from bacteria to animals, including humans.

Manganese

Manganese is an essential trace mineral in animal nutrition and is believed to be an essential trace mineral in human nutrition, as well. Manganese is a metallic element with atomic number 25 and an atomic weight of 54.94 daltons. Its chemical symbol is Mn. Dietary manganese deficiency in animals results in a wide variety of structural and physiological defects, including growth retardation, skeletal and cartilage malformations, impaired reproductive function, congenital ataxia due to abnormal inner ear development, optic nerve abnormalities, impaired insulin metabolism and abnormal glucose tolerance, alterations in lipoprotein metabolism and an impaired oxidant defense system. The richest dietary sources of manganese include whole grains, nuts, leafy vegetables and teas. Manganese is concentrated in the bran of grains which is removed during processing.

Copper

Copper is an essential trace mineral in animal and human nutrition. Anemia, neutropenia and osteoporosis are found with frank copper deficiency. Copper deficiency in humans is rare but it does occur under certain circumstances, such as in patients receiving long-term total parenteral nutrition (TPN). Mild copper deficiency due to marginal copper intake over a long period may also occur. In addition to possible anemia, neutropenia and osteoporosis, manifestations of mild copper deficiency may include abnormal glucose tolerance, hypercholesterolemia, arthritis, myocardial disease, arterial disease, cardiac arrhythmias, loss of pigmentation and neurological problems.

Zinc

Zinc is an essential element in human and animal nutrition with a wide range of biological roles. Zinc plays catalytic, structural or regulatory roles in the more than 200 zinc metalloenzymes that have been identified in biological systems. These enzymes are involved in nucleic acid and protein metabolism and the production of energy, among other things. Zinc plays a structural role in the formation of the so-called zinc fingers. Zinc fingers are exploited by transcription factors for interacting with DNA and regulating the activity of genes. Another structural role of zinc is in the maintenance of the integrity of biological membranes resulting in their protection against oxidative injury, among other things.

Sodium

Sodium is sodium chloride or table salt a mineral, one of a very few rocks commonly eaten by humans. There are different forms of edible salt: unrefined salt, refined salt, table salt or iodised salt. It is a crystalline solid, white, pale pink or light grey in colour, obtained from sea water or rock deposits. In nature, it includes not only sodium chloride, but also other vital trace minerals.Salt is necessary for the survival of all living creatures, including humans. Salt is involved in regulating the water content (fluid balance) of the body. Salt flavour is one of the basic tastes. Salt cravings may be caused by trace mineral deficiencies as well as by a deficiency of sodium chloride itself. Salt is required for life, but overconsumption can increase the risk of health problems, including high blood pressure, in those individuals who are genetically predisposed to hypertension.

Selenium

Selenium is an essential trace element in human and animal nutrition. It is involved in the defense against the toxicity of reactive oxygen species, in the regulation of thyroid hormone metabolism and the regulation of the redox state of cells. The amount of selenium in food is a function of the selenium content of the soil. Selenium enters the food chain through incorporation into plant proteins as the amino acids L-selenocysteine and L-selenomethionine. Selenium, like most trace elements and minerals, is not evenly distributed in the world's soil.

Potassium

Potassium is an essential macromineral in human nutrition with a wide range of biochemical and physiological roles. Among other things, it is important in the transmission of nerve impulses, the contraction of cardiac, skeletal and smooth muscle, the production of energy, the synthesis of nucleic acids, the maintenance of intracellular tonicity and the maintenance of normal blood pressure. Accumulating evidence suggests that diets high in potassium may be protective not only against hypertension, but also strokes and cardiovascular disease and possibly other degenerative diseases, as well.

Phosphorous

Phosphorus is an essential macromineral in human nutrition and plays pivotal roles in the structure and function of the body. Phosphorus is essential for the process of bone mineralization and makes up the structure of bone. Approximately 85 per cent of phosphorus in the adult body is in bone. Phosphorus in the form of phospholipids makes up the structure of cellular membranes. Phosphorus also makes up the structure of nucleic acids and nucleotides, including adenosine triphosphate, among other things. Life has been said to be built around phosphorus.

Magnesium

Magnesium is an essential mineral in human nutrition with a wide range of biological functions. Magnesium is involved in over 300 metabolic reactions. It is necessary for every major biological process, including the production of cellular energy and the synthesis of nucleic acids and proteins. It is also important for the electrical stability of cells, the maintenance of membrane integrity, muscle contraction, nerve conduction and the regulation of vascular tone, among other things.

Magnesium is an alkaline earth metal with atomic number 12 and an atomic weight of 24.31 daltons. Its chemical symbol is Mg. The total body magnesium content of an adult is about 25 grams. About 50 per cent -60 per cent exists in bone. Magnesium is the second most abundant intracellular cation; potassium is the most abundant.

As opined by Karen Bartlett the cell salts have serious characteristics in conjunction with the unique process known as spagyrics and it's role in human therapeutics.

Cell salts are homeopathic preparations of certain mineral compounds found within all living things. Cell salts represent a self contained homeopathic system that lends itself to use as nutritional supplement.

Twelve in number, cell salts are an extremely versatile, natural healing method. This system of Medicine is based upon the "cell theory" of Virchow in 1858. He said that the body is a collection of cells and that all medical treatment should center around the health of the individual cell. Together with Schuessler, they developed a system of medicine based on cellular health.

In 1873, German biochemist, William H. Schuessler found that there are certain essential minerals that the body requires. He discovered this by studying the remains of numerous cadavers and examining them after calcinations or burning to see what essential elements remained. Schuessler found that according to the time of year we are born we are deficient in three of the cell salts. Replenishing that deficiency through micro cell nutrients greatly improves the health of the body.

It was also found as well that the cell salts provide remedies for many illnesses, not as a medicine, but as an enhancer for the health of the body on a cell level, helping the body to heal itself.

He found that an imbalance or a lack of any of these minerals may lead to disease in the tissues so lacking. Providing the missing minerals to the tissues corrects that imbalance and so eliminates the illness.

Thus the cell salts provide a rebalancing of the body enabling its natural disease controlling mechanisms to function. To this end, the cell salts are not a "cure" or a medicine per se but a body function balancing supplement albeit a powerful one nonetheless.

The importance of the inorganic components of cells were recognized, hence the 12 salts were found to be the basic building blocks of the cell and water and other organic substances were used by the salts in building the cells of the body.

If there is a deficiency in any of these salts the cell and consequently the body would suffer.

Charles W. Littlefield, analytical chemist, wrote:

"The twelve mineral salts are, in a very real sense, the material basis of the organs and tissues of the body and are absolutely essential to their integrity of structure and functional activity. Experiments prove that the various tissue salts will rapidly disintegrate in the absence of the proper proportion of these salts in the circulation fluid. Whereas the maintenance of this proportion insures healthy growth and perpetual renewal.

These mineral salts are, therefore, the physical basis of all healing. Regardless of the school employed, if these are absent from the blood and tissues, no permanent cure is possible."

These 12 salts are essential for the health and growth of the body. They are grouped in fours; Phosphates, Chlorides, Sulphates, and Fluorides (also Silica).

The 12 salts are as follows; Calcium Phosphate, Ferrum Phosphate, Kali Phosphate, Natrum Phosphate, Kali Mur., Natrum Mur, Calcium Sulph, Natrum Sulph, Kali Sulph, Calcium Fluor., and Silica.

These 12 salts were found to make up the human body.

Due to the minute scale of cells, the ideal way to replenish any deficiency is through very small micronutrients that go directly to the depleted cells.

Tinctures of the salts provide an easily absorbed transport for the body, enabling the needed salts to go directly to the bloodstream without the body expending much needed energy in digesting and processing the micronutrient cell salts.

According to Robert Bartlett Our cells are replaced cyclically on a regular basis. When the cell does not have the proper materials that it needs to be a healthy cell, our overall health suffers. Cell Salts provide the components that our cells need to be healthy. Taken on a regular basis over a period of time our cells rebuild themselves with the proper healthy materials that we need.

All our internal organs; our skin, our blood, all made up of cells. The health of our body is dependent upon the health of the smallest part of our body; the cell. These Salt level extracts contain the spagyric essence, which is made by purifying the plant or mineral body until it becomes a clear or white crystalline salt, and then adding the salt to the alcohol tincture to capture the physical signatures of the plant or mineral. This part of the extract serves to give the essence "body" in alchemical terms and helps to carry its healing actions into the physical.

According to Kristine Danowski, ancient alchemy combined both the practical and the mystical. Practical chemistry included metallurgy (mining and purification of metals for weaponry, jewelry, and coins), art (paints, inks, dyes), medicine (various healing herbs and herbal preparations, funeral rites), and the mundane (flavoring herbs, spices, cosmetics). For example, ancient texts describe metallurgical methods that, when followed as written, produce quantitative yields of nearly pure metals.

Civilizations depended on these metals, so naturally they would know how to extract and purify them. Mystical chemistry was the search for the Philosopher's Stone, symbolism, and various theories about the origin of matter.

Many of our chronic diseases are actually caused due to excessive inflammation. Inflammation is initiated by the neutrophils, it's granules release cytotoxic metabolites aimed at destroying microbials and viral invaders, and by basophils to destroy allergens. Cytotoxic metabolites include peroxides and free radicals, these oxidising elements can also destroy the fatty acids that comprise cell membranes, causing necrosis of tissues in the inflammated area, their over activity is suppressed by anti oxdidants produced by the cells. Anti-oxidants include the enzymes, vitamins A, E and C, zinc, copper and selenium, hence, these elements are required for the immune system or body's defence mechanism, the inflammatory attack and the healing of tissues. The special aspect of the ancient technique followed in preparation of Spagyric Medicines is that importance is given to the mineral salts which are present in the plants grown in their natural habitats, as plants grown in different enviornments usually show a wide variation of mineral salt composition.

For instance, a plant grown in limestone soil would be expected to have a higher calcium content in comparison to the same plant grown in sandy soil. Analysis carried out by German and British Scientists has shown the presence of mineral salts like iron, calcium, sodium, sulphar, etc. and trace elements like zinc, potassium, copper, cobalt, selenium, magnesium and manganese in the medicinal plants.

The following is a quote from a book by a distinguished French Scientist Professor C. Louis Kervran (1901-1983) who has been nominated for the 1975 Nobel Prize in Physiology; "Classical agriculture (by this I mean the science that is taught in schools), is a huge imposture, which is frightening in its cynicism. It recommends the use of complete fertilizers, the word "complete" being identified with 'N' 'P' and 'K', as if these three elements were the only ones to be found in plants. Its basic postulate is to restore in quality and quantity, the soil's elements taken from it by the yearly harvest. One may say that this agriculture has enclosed itself in a dilemma:

A. If the law of restitution is to be satisfied (whereby one implicitly recognizes that elements other than N, P, and K are taken away at harvest), the plant would have to find these other elements in the soil in limitless amounts.

B. Or, plants themselves must make these elements found at harvest and not provided for by the soil. Implicit in this alternative, is a transmutation of elements through a biological channel."

The founders of the Agricultural Research Station at Rothamstead, Lawes and Gilbert, in a series of classic experiments, found that plants appeared to extract more elements from the soil, than the soil actually contained.

In 1873, the analytic chemist, Albrecht von Herzeele, published a book entitled "The Origin of Inorganic Substances" which offered proof that plants transmute the elements, for example, Phosphorous into Sulphur, Calcium into Phosphorous, Magnesium into Calcium, Carbonic acid into Magnesium and Nitrogen.

Professor Hisatoki Komaki, an agronomist at the Institute for Biological Agriculture (Otsu, Japan), presented a paper entitled: 'Observations on Non-Radioactive Biological Cold Fusion, Using Saccharomyces Cerevisiae', at the seventh International Conference on Cold Fusion in 1998 (Yeast of the sugar fungi tribe).The paper describes how Komaki and his team performed a number of carefully controlled experiments, and were able to successfully verify that certain types of fungus can create iron and magnesium, by transmuting other elements.

All life forms are mineral based. Nearly all life forms depend upon the green plants for sustenance, irrespective of whether they are herbivore or carnivore. The major difference between a molecule of chlorophyll and a molecule of blood, is in the central atom of those respective molecules.

For chlorophyll, it is magnesium, and for blood it is iron. The human body has a poor tolerance for crude minerals, with many having extremely toxic effects. As a general example, if iron is prescribed for anaemia, it is invariably a preparation of the crude metal. Many generation of women can attest to its constipating effect and the subsequent resort to laxatives.

However, if the iron has been Bio-chelated (passed through a plant), then it is readily assimilated by the body with none of the side effects.

Deficiency of minerals causes a disorder to the normal function of the organism. Calcium deficiency causes osteomalacia, cardiac disorders, and neuromuscular excitability. Potassium deficiency causes cardiac dysfunction and disorders of the acid-base equilibrium. Sodium deficiency causes withholding or loss of water of the organism. Iodine deficiency causes goiter. Magnesium deficiency causes neuromuscular disorders, cardiac dysfunction and osteomalacia. Ferrum deficiency causes anemia. Zinc deficiency causes dermatological disorders, dysfunction of retina, diabetes, azoospermia, abortion, senility. Copper deficiency causes hepatolenticular degeneration, osteoporosis, and anemia. Cobalt deficiency causes anemia and general weakness. Selenium deficiency causes muscular dystrophy and cardiac dysfunction.

Nobel Prize Winner for Bio-Chemistry, Linus Pauling PhD., considered that a mineral deficiency was the foremost predisposing factor in the genesis of disease within the body. Analysis of the cremated remains of the human body, has shown that the remains consist primarily of 12 different salts, as follows:

1. Calcium phosphate
2. Calcium sulphate
3. Calcium fluoride
4. Potassium phosphate
5. Potassium sulphate
6. Potassium chloride
7. Sodium phosphate
8. Sodium sulphate
9. Sodium sulphate
10. Sodium sulphate
11. Magnesium phosphate
12. Silicon dioxide

There is a very effective system of therapy based upon those salts, which was devised by a German homoeopathic physician,

Wilhelm Schüssler. It is important to remember that single salt, or combinations of them, as found in plants, will act on the cellular level. However the salts are strongly alkaline and must never be used except in Homoeopathic potencies. An orthodox extract or tincture will only operate on the organ level, for the simple reason that they do not contain all of the bio-chelated cell salts, and thus, must be considered incomplete extracts. Whereas, the Spagyric method produces a complete extraction of the plant. In Homoeopathy minerals are used in accordance with the principles developed by German homoeopathic physician, Wilhelm Schüssler (1822-1898). Schüssler reasoned that since the remains of the human body, when it is burned to ashes, primarily consist of 12 mineral salts, listed above, these minerals must play a vital role in the body's integrity and function. In addition, the different organs and parts of the body in turn reveal different combinations of minerals. Schüssler's method consisted of administering the appropriate minerals to correct deficiencies, which he identified in his patients using a complex diagnostic system, and as Physiologists have established salt-hunger or 'Chelation' causes ailments in human beings, The majority of mineral salts are soluble in water not in alcohol, so, even from the modern scientific view Plant Alchemy is totally scientific in which mineral salts produced in and from natural sources (in Biochemistry chemically produced mineral salts are used throughout) in minute form is prescribed to relieve mineral salt defficiency or 'Chelation' in human body, thus to effect a far more natural and specific Cure.

8

Alchemy and the Zodiac Connection

Spagyric processing results in medicines with are both natural and pure, with a full spectrum of healing qualities on all levels of being.

There are two principles active in man; one is the principle of Matter, the other one is the Spirit. The Spirit in man sustains the body as the air supplies him with life. - ***Paracelsus*** -

The material organism derives all sensation and performs all functions of life solely by means of the immaterial being- the vital force. - ***Hahnemann*** -

As a magnet may induce magnetism in a bar of iron, a plant may induce certain vital powers to become active in certain organs.

- ***Franz Hartmann, MD*** -

These writings express the ancient idea that all beings, whether mineral, animal, or plant, are animated by an inner vital life force.

This vital force has been called by many names, including Prana, Qi, and Spirit, and its study has continued as an unbroken thread from ancient Oriental, Ayurvedic, and Alchemical healing through the more recent systems of Homeopathy, Oriental medicine, and the Energy medicine tradition.

Alchemists believed that we are surrounded by the material world we live in it and actively operate on it. We are also its prisoner. The world dictates what and how we do. Alchemists, though they be in any country and any age, seeking the means to capture experience from this material world to escape. We see the evolution of the alchemy of art, and alchemy itself is based on five postulates:

1. The entire universe is divine in origin and nature.
2. All organisms, no matter how fine or coarse, contain within the divine spark of life and are interconnected with one another.
3. All organisms are in a state of constant development and its synthesis continues to perfection.
4. People are part of the universe. They therefore have a divine origin and by their actions or inaction affect all organisms in all spheres of being.
5. People can that understand the basic laws that govern the one hand, their being on the other side of the universe, learn to recognize the divine spark of life energy in all organisms, isolate it, it purification and manipulate it so as to accelerate process of evolution.

Note that there was no word of any transformation of matter, the artificial person or immortality. There is talk here about the Almighty, the basic principle of the universe, and man as a kind of synthesizer. It is assumed here that one can identify themselves through knowledge seemed suddenly as if the only knowledge of a violent attack, align with the principles of the universe, the principles of creation. But then everything else, such as the conversion of anything in anything else, such as immortality, there is little impact of this major intersection. This of course leads to reflection on the relationship of alchemy and science. We are tempted to identify one with another. Alchemy also interferes with natural processes in order to discover principles. The same does science.

Alchemy can be considered from various perspectives. It is certainly possible to become an alchemist, and many people went and still goes this way. Is it possible to examine the historical, dealing with the creation, development and changes in the alchemy of time and its various manifestations, as occurred in various places around the globe. It can be interpreted - by the way went to Carl Gustav Jung. This took the symbolism of the alchemists, in particular those based on the symbolism of male and female principles. Jung in his interpretation tried to infer that alchemy was essentially a mystical protopsychologií. According to his conception of the alchemists were engaged in physical subject matter, but at the core they were developing themselves, concentrating on the mental process of discovery and self-awareness. And of course it can conceive of inspiration, as the source of the story, as an ancient, holistic nature cures the Spagyric body, mind and soul, considered as a unit in equilibrium.

Alchemy is characterised into three broad disciplines, Metal Alchemy, Biological Alchemy and Spagyrics or Plant Alchemy. Spagyric the preparation of plant is keen that the plant be used by all three principles (body, mind and soul) and represented in the finished tincture in a balanced ratio. Spagyric will never isolate individual compounds from the plant. By spagyric treatment is the healing power will be increased and the patient as a whole benefit. Spagyric medicine is an ancient natural system of healing and has been brought up to date using modern pharmaceutical methods of manufacture and safety standards.

Derived entirely from plants, each individual spagyric essence is made from a particular plant, its healing power increased by Spagyric transformation. The word "Spagyric" comes from two Greek words meaning "to separate or purify" and "to reunite", alluding to the specific preparation process of a Spagyric essence. Given to a patient, such a remedy mobilises his/her self-healing forces. Paracelsus, the great 16th century Swiss healer brought medicine and alchemy together to create his own method. He strongly believed in the connection between humankind and nature and that plants were placed on Earth for our benefit. To Paracelsus is attributed the Doctrine of Signatures: the concept that the healing potential of a plant is shown in its very form, or "signature". Plants are natural remedies and their healing power can be increased by Spagyric transformation.

Astrology

Astrology is likely one of the most misunderstood aspects of esoteric philosophy, often seen as mere fortune telling. In reality, astrology- like the other aspects of the Organic Unity paradigm, is based on direct observation of nature. Its roots go back to ancient India and Mesopotamia, and is considered the sister science to alchemy. Whether one believes in astrology or not, the fact remains that it has been a part of numerous cultures from around the world for thousands of years and that it works regardless of the system of used. Systems do not stick around for thousands of years if they lack validity. The two practical uses of astrology within this system are for the preparation of medicinal substances and for specific evaluation of ones health.

As for the preparation of plant medicines, astrology teaches about proper timing. Thus, the plant is able to be harvested, prepared, and utilized in a way that is harmonious with the plants own energetic constitution. For example, if one has a plant ruled by the Sun, it would be harvested and processed on Sunday at the Sun hour, thus exalting that energetic component of the plant. This would make the remedy more specific for a persons own inner Sun, being the heart and overall vitality. Astrology allows for correspondences and connections to be made between a plant, a person, and the cosmos.

It was common practice for herbalist in the ancient times to have a thorough understanding of the stars in order to properly align their medicines with their celestial counterpart, as well as effectively diagnose and treat their patients. The natal chart can be used as a tool to understand the preconditioned strengths and weaknesses of ones being (constitution/temperament) and thus the energetic architecture that determines how and when they will get sick.

The three modes of astrology correspond with the three principles of alchemy, the three worlds of the shaman, and the three doshas of Ayurveda. The four elements of Astrology are the same within all of the systems. The seven planets are a more complex expression of the pattern of existence: Sun, Moon, Mercury, Mars, Venus, Saturn and Jupiter. Whereas the four elements provide the energetics of a particular season, the planets provide a more refined picture of the pattern at play in nature. The twelve archetypes or signs, give further specificity. Each level or dimension is a different lens of perception, and gives different layers of information.

Peter Morrell postulated that, there are seven metals in the ancient alchemical system of healing, which have resurfaced from time to time in medical thought, these are:

1. Gold
2. Silver
3. Mercury
4. Copper
5. Iron
6. Tin
7. Lead

These metals correspond respectively to the planets sun, moon, mercury, venus, mars, jupiter and saturn. These in turn correspond with certain key qualities or personalities described in detail in astrology and Hermetic science. Stated simplistically and for brevity, mars is seen as masculine and active, venus is feminine, artistic and passive, jupiter the theorizer, saturn the lord of death, mercury the communicator, sun the day-king and moon the night goddess.

They are also deemed to correspond to the parts of the body as follows:

Sun-gold-aurum-	heart and spine
Moon-silver-argentum-	brain and fluids
Mercury-mercury-hydrargyrum-	nervous system, lungs
Venus-copper-cuprum-	kidneys, nutrition
Mars-iron-ferrum-	blood, muscles and circulation
Jupiter-tin-stannum-	liver and gall bladder
Saturn-lead-plumbum-	skeleton and skin, hair, nails

Similarly the planets and metals correspond to certain colours. There are various schemes. One such scheme is as follows:

Sun-gold-	golds, yellows
Moon-silver-	white, cream, greens
Mercury-mercury-	silver, grey, yellow
Venus-copper-	blues, pinks, pastel shades
Mars-iron-	reds and browns
Jupiter-tin-	oranges
Saturn-lead-	black, dark colours, purple, violet, indigo

Because foods can also be classified as the seven metals, one may change one's diet so as to reduce foods that are harmful for you and increase your use of more helpful foods. This applies generally, not just to considerations of which foods might be rich in which metals. Some food correspondences are shown:

Sun-	sunflower seeds, oranges, eggs, grapes
Moon-	melons, cucumbers, yogurt, cheese, milk
Mercury-	cereals
Venus-	fruits, potato, chocolate, sweets, berries
Mars-	peppers, tomatoes, onion, garlic, curry, meats, black pudding
Jupiter-	nuts, seeds, lemons, apples
Saturn-	coffee, carob, aubergenes, olives

Alchemy and The Zodiac Connection

Aires	*Calcination*	2,3,4 *Wands*
Taurus	*Congealation*	5,6,7 *Pentacles*
Gemini	*Fixation*	8,9,10 *Swords*
Leo	*Digestion*	2,3,4 *Cups*
Virgo	*Distillation*	8,9,10 *Pentacles*
Libra	*Sublimation*	2,3,4 *Swords*
Scorpio	*Putrefaction*	5,6,7 *Cups*
Saggitarious	*Incineration*	8,9,10 *Wands*
Capricorn	*Fermentation*	2,3,4 *Pentacles*
Aquarious	*Dissolution*	5,6,7 *Swords*
Pisces	*Projection*	8,9,10 *Cups*

Alchemical and spagyric philosophy works with the same planetary archetypes found in Qabala and astrology, as seen in the familiar diagram of the Tree of Life. As in Qabala, each planetary sphere has individual qualities associated with it, such as deities, colours, musical tones, and days of the week. In spagyric work, each of these planets also rules organs, organ systems, and body parts, diseases and healing effects, and herbs. This rulership is a two-way interaction called *sympathy*, and refers to the planetary energies from above affecting beings below, and the beings below manifesting different proportions of these planetary energies. These sympathies, as ruled by each planet, can also be organized according to the planets, using the celestial archetypes as a sort of filing cabinet for easily structuring and understanding otherwise scattered pieces of healing and herbal knowledge.

The first concepts to examine in order to use this system, then, are the individual planets, their energies, and rulerships. "As above, so below" means that, like the universe, each living being is made up of diverse individual parts. In the universe, these parts are the planets, moving in their orbits, affecting each other in structured and predictable ways. In the living beings on earth, these parts are organs and body parts, each performing its function, and, like the planets, each able to affect any of the others. Some of the living beings on earth, such as plants, manufacture chemicals in themselves which can affect the organs and health of other beings, this, too, follows the same planetary sympathies.

By developing an understanding of these sympathies and their interactions with each other, we can easily work to rectify the energetic imbalances that can lead to illness, and can also work to strengthen particular energies within ourselves for physical or spiritual improvement.

Moon

The Moon is the first planet we will discuss. The Moon is cyclical, and changes in a regular and repeated way, affecting the waters of the earth with its changes. Cycles and water are the prominent aspects of the Moon's medical rulership as well. Any rhythmic or cyclical events of the body's function, as well as the fluids of the body, are all ruled by the Moon. This includes cycles such as the circadian rhythms or menstrual cycle, and the fluids of the glands and stomach. The Moon's organs are the stomach and brain, the womb, and the glandular and hormonal system. On the more subtle levels, the Moon rules the emotions, the astral body, and the subconscious.

Illnesses affecting any of the Moon's organs or systems would be considered Lunar ailments, such as stomachaches, headaches or emotional illnesses. The Moon also rules problems of the brain which are related to structure, such as tumors. Some other good examples of Lunar disorders are seasonal depression, which is both emotional and cyclical, and pre-menstrual syndrome, which is both hormonal and emotional.

Some effects common to herbs of the Moon are sedative, hormone-balancing, tonic to the brain or stomach, and narcotic or pain killing. Many nutritious vegetables are ruled by the Moon, as are plants which are cooling or moisturizing cucumber is a Lunar plant exhibiting all of these properties. Lunar herbs are also marked by an either rotten or sweet to sickly sweet smell, as with Valerian root or Jasmine.

Mars

Mars was named after the god of war, and its attributes fall within that archetype. Mars rules aggression, the will, determination, passion, and the survival instinct. Physically, Mars rules the blood, especially the iron component, the immune system (the body's army of defense), the sexual organs and drive, and the adrenal glands.

Mars rules injuries and accidents, as well as blood and immuno-deficiency diseases. A simple, overall picture of Mars' rulership can be seen if we think of Mars as a heating, stimulating, and tensing influence. This influence can lead to problems such as fevers, rashes, infections, and the various illnesses from stress and aggression, such as anger or violence, hypertension and ulcers. While these problems may initially seem diverse and unrelated, all of them arise from one or more of Mars' qualities of heat, stimulation, or tension.

Mars herbs tend to be forceful, stimulating, heating, and cleansing or purgative. Mars herbs are often used to detoxify the system and nourish the blood, and many contain large amounts of iron. Mars can also be used to give more force to other aspects of treatment. Mars herbs often have sharp, hot, or pungent smells and tastes, such as Cayenne. They may also be prickly or have stinging defenses, such as Nettle, which is high in iron, and a classic herb of Mars.

Mercury

In mythology, Mercury is the swift messenger, and in chemistry, is a slippery, changeable fluid metal. The planet Mercury, which is a fast-moving planet and one which frequently changes direction, was aptly named. Mercury rules quickness, speech, cleverness, thought, and the mind, or function of the brain. Mercury also rules writing, communication, intelligence and reasoning. Physically, Mercury rules the electrical activity of the body, in the brain and nerves, as well as the lungs and throat. The life force and vitality in general are also ruled by Mercury.

Mercury rules problems of these organs and systems, such as lung disease, nerve disorders, and problems of the brain which are related to function, such as Alzheimer's disease. On the more subtle levels, Mercury is often a factor in both dyslexia and stuttering, which are both disorders of communication, the first incoming, the second outgoing. Autism reflects Mercury's imbalance in both directions, as do many other cognitive and behavioural problems.

Many herbs which are non-specifically balancing, or adaptogenic, are ruled by Mercury, as would be herbs affecting the activity of the brain or nerves, or the lungs and throat. Mercury herbs tend to have very aromatic scents, often very pleasant but not long-lasting. Lavender is an example of a Mercury herb, used in aromatherapy for balancing the emotions, whether stimulation or calming is needed. Another signature of Mercury herbs is a licorice-like flavour, which is often associated with hormone-balancing activity. Some examples of this are Licorice (which is also used for the lungs and throat), Anise, or Fennel.

Jupiter

Jupiter is expansive in quality, and the root of the word "jovial", and rules the personality qualities of generosity, selflessness, and cheerfulness. In the body, Jupiter rules the liver, the metabolism, the anabolic and building processes of the body, nourishment of the body from food, and the fatty tissues. Jupiter also rules judgement, which can mean the digestive organ's judgements about assimilating or rejecting food, or the more intellectual forms of personal judgement.

Jupiter illnesses can be those affecting the liver or digestive systems, or the more subtle disorders which arise from poor judgement, such as overeating. Since Jupiter also rules over-indulgence, alcoholism is a good example of a Jupiter disease, arising from a personal choice to ingest harmful amounts of alcohol, which eventually affects the liver.

The herbs ruled by Jupiter tend to be general, supportive or nutritive tonics, and are often stimulating to appetite, digestion, and weight gain. Jupiter also rules laxative herbs and herbs which aid or protect the liver. A bright yellow colour and bitter taste are common to many of these herbs, Turmeric being a good example.

Venus

The archetype of love and beauty, Venus also rules refinement and the arts. Venus rules the true love of friendship and affection which transcends the sexual energies, and resides in the heart chakra or center. Medically, Venus rules the kidneys and urinary system and the skin, especially the face.

Besides the physical illnesses which affect the skin and kidneys, Venus rules many subtle or emotionally-related conditions. Many skin problems are aggravated by emotional upset, and this encompasses Venus's energy on two levels. Venus's influence can also be seen whenever the heart is affected by emotional states. Heart palpitations or fainting in response to intense emotion is one way this can manifest; fainting at weddings is a classic example. Venus also rules any chronic depressive states involving love or emotion, such as the inability to overcome the loss of a loved one. Also, since the realm of Venus is one of refinement and beauty and may be more pleasant than the real world, those who are emotionally escapist or lost in illusions often have an imbalance of Venus energy.

The therapeutic effects of Venus herbs are toning and astringent to the skin, cleansing and supportive to the kidneys and urinary system, and aphrodisiac or balancing to the female system or hormones. Venus herbs are generally very sweet in smell and taste, but not in the excessive way that Moon herbs are. Venus also rules many fruit-bearing plants, such as cherries, strawberries, and pears. Rose is the most archetypal expression of Venus energy, and is beautiful and sweet-smelling, used for its astringent effects and its balancing action on the female system, and also valued for its fruit, rosehips.

Saturn

In mythical literature, Saturn is also Chronos, the father of time. In astrology, Saturn is a cold planet of restriction and limitation, and the dispenser of karma and fate. Some of the other characteristics that come from Saturn's influence are diplomacy, the work ethic, and self-control. Physically, Saturn rules the spleen and all of the structural tissues of the body, such as the bones and teeth.

Saturn rules any diseases of the spleen or bones, as well as any structural weaknesses of the body. Also ruled by Saturn are all slow, chronic processes such as aging. Osteoporosis and arthritis are good examples of multi-level Saturn diseases, arising with age and affecting the bones. Many of the same problems which are ruled by Mars, such as hypertension, ulcers, or heart problems, can also be caused by Saturn's influence. The difference is that, while Mars gives rise to these problems through its driving influence of aggression, Saturn's influence can cause the same stresses in those who feel an overwhelming need to control the situations around them. A serious imbalance of Saturn can even lead to the severe emotional states seen in many phobias or obsessive-compulsive disorders, which often arise from a fear of losing control.

Saturn herbs tend to be extremely shrinking and drying, much more than Venus's gentle astringents, and also can be mineralizing or supportive to the bones and hard tissues. Comfrey is an herb of Saturn which is used for treating broken bones and mineral deficiencies, and was anciently called Knitbone. The leaves of Comfrey are so covered in fine but stiff hairs as to feel dry, like sandpaper, but not prickly like a Mars herb might be. Any herbs used for the spleen would also be ruled by Saturn, as are many poisonous herbs. The energy of Saturn can also be used to affect other aspects of therapy by determining them to the more physical plane.

Sun

The Sun is the center of our universe, and appropriately rules the self, the ego and individuality, as well as creative masculine energy and vitality. The Sun rules charisma or the lack of it, and how we present ourselves to others. Just as the Sun circulates warmth and life through the universe, its organ, the heart, circulates warmth and life through the body. The Sun, giving light to the earth, also rules vision and the eyes.

The Sun rules any heart problems which are of a functional or structural nature, as well as circulatory problems and eye disorders. The Sun also rules self-esteem problems, and often Sun herbs are helpful with anorexia, which is a disorder arising both from lack of self-esteem and from a misunderstanding of other's perceptions of you. The Sun's influence can also be connected with substance abuse, if it is occurring as a form of self-destruction due to low self-esteem, rather than Jupiter's over-indulgence and poor judgement.

Solar herbs are those used to support the eyes, heart, and circulation, and also used as general tonics and male aphrodisiacs. Solar herbs are warming, and often have very pungent or warm scents, but are not as strongly hot as Mars herbs. Some examples are Ginger or Rosemary, which both have pleasantly warm smells and are used to warm the body and increase circulation, but are not nearly as hot as Mars' cayenne.

Once the archetypal energies and the healing attributes they rule are understood, one can begin to both use this knowledge and add to it. As health issues are examined and addressed, the planetary system can be used as a guide to treatment. And, as more knowledge about herbs and health is gained, this new knowledge can be integrated into the planetary framework.

This planetary framework thus just a structural system many illnesses have one planetary rulership in their action, but affect an organ of another rulership. Even within one organ there may be different influences, such as the Moon ruling the brain's tissue and structure, but Mercury ruling its function and activity.

Herbs, too, can be ambiguous, and the examples we have given above are intended only to illustrate an overall pattern that is the real system. Every medicinal herb has more than one effect. Sometimes, all effects are clearly under one ruler, sometimes they are diverse and seemingly contradictory. Nicholas Culpeper gives a good example of this in his book, originally written in the early 17th century. Discussing blackberries as ruled by Venus because they bear fruit, he asks why the plant is so prickly. His answer is that they are under Venus, but here she is in Mars' house of Aries. The possibility of such a dual rulership is another factor to consider in selecting herbs for particular effects.

The variations in energy are an opening for the use of the alchemical Art. A plant which exhibits a few different attributes can be worked with alchemically and spagyrically to magnify one quality over another, or to work on one level of being more than another. Rather than being a source of confusion, the complexities of this system should be seen as an opportunity to apply important practical aspects of alchemical and spagyric work, such as planetary timing and spiritual interaction with the laboratory operations.

This is why the overall pattern should be understood deeply, so that every person using the system feels confident enough to apply their knowledge in the way that suits them best. Instead of consulting ten different books and getting ten different answers for a plant's rulership or usefulness for a certain planetary condition, each of us should be able to understand the individual nature of both plant and medicine, and to apply that understanding in a personal way, which may or may not agree with other people's usage.

There are a few approaches for working with planetary healing. The most simple is to use the planetary energies themselves to support organs, systems, or functions of the body or to oppose disorders, all according to planetary rulership. Using Mars herbs to boost the immune system is an example of the supportive approach; an example of the opposing energies technique would be the use of a skin-toning, cleansing, astringent herb of Venus to treat a hot, inflamed rash, ruled by Mars, Venus's opposite.

Plants and their Corresponding Planets

Plants which are subject to particularly the Jupiter

Pimpernel (Anagallis arvensis)

Maple (Acer campestre)

Elecampane (Inula campana)

Alexandrian parsley (Smyrnium olusatrum)

Anis (Pimpinella anisum) (with Mercury)

Apple tree (Pirus malus)

Apricot tree (Prunus armeniaca)

Arnica (Arnica montana)

Basil (Ocimum basilicum) (with Mars)

Comfrey (Symphytum officinale)

Blueberry (Vaccinium myrtillus)

Borage (Borrago officinalis)

Chestnut (Castanea sativa) (with Venus)

Marshmallow (Althaea officinalis) (with sun and Venus)

Oak (Quercus robur) (with Mars)

Endive (Cichorium endive)

Polypody (Polypodium vulgare)

Engelsüß Fumitory (Fumaria officinalis)

Ash (Fraxinus excelsior) (with sun)

Madder (Rubia tinctorum)

Fig tree (Ficus carica) (with Venus)

Fennel (Foeniculum vulgare) (with Mercury)

Cinquefoil (Potentilla reptans)

Garden chervil (Anthriscus cerefolium)

Yellow gentian (Gentiana lutea) (with sun)

Ginseng (Panax ginseng)

Large-flowered mullein (Verbascum thapsiforme)

Oats (Avena sativa) (with Mercury)
Sempervivum (Sempervivum tectorum)
Dog Rose (Rosa canina) (with Mars)
Raspberry (Rubus idaeus)
Coltsfoot (Tussilago farfara) (with Mercury)
Dog grass (Agropyron caninum)
Iceland moss (Cetraria islandica)
Jasmine (Jasminum officinale)
Lavender (Lavandula vera) (with Mercury and Sun)
Liverwort (Marchantia polymorpha)
Lebermoosart (Liverworts, various Species)
Hepaticae (Anemone hepatica)
Linseed/flax (Linum usitatissimum) (with Saturn and Mars)
Linde (Tilia europaea) (with Venus)
Laurel (Laurus nobilis) (with sun)
Dandelion (Taraxacum officinale)
Lungwort (Pulmonaria officinalis) (with Mercury)
Almond (Prunus dulcis) (with Sun)
Amygdalum (Amygdalum polytum)
Manna (Fraxinus ornus)
Meisterwurz (Imperatoria ostruthium)
Lemon balm (Melissa officinalis) (with Sun)
Mistletoe (Viscum album) (with Sun and Moon)
Nutmeg tree (Myristica fragrans) (with Moon)
Myrrh (Commiphora myrrha) (with Sun)
Carnation (Dianthus cariophyllus)
Agrimony (Agrimonia eupatoria)
Olive tree (Olea europaea) (with Sun)
Poplar (Populus species) (with Saturn and Sun)
Peppermint (Mentha piperita) (with Venus)

Tansy (Tanacetum vulgare)

Rose (Rosa damascena) (with Venus)

Horse chestnut (Aesculus hippocastanum)

Red sandalwood (Santalum rubrum) (with Venus)

Sage (Salvia officinalis)

Sorrel (Rumex acetosa)

Celandine (Chelidonium majus) (with Sun)

Black henbane (Hyoscyamus niger) (With Saturn and Neptune)

Asparagus (Asparagus officinalis)

Sweet clover (Melilotus officinalis)

Licorice (Liquiritiae officinalis/Glycyrrhiza glabra) (with Mercury)

Centaury (Centaurium umbellatum)

Tomato (Solanum lycopersicum)

Juniper (Juniperus communis) (with Sun and Mercury)

Chicory (Cichorium intybus)

Grapevine (Vitis vinifera) (with Sun)

White sandalwood (Santalum album) (with Venus)

Hyssop (Hyssopus officinalis) (with Moon and Mars)

Betony (Betonica officinalis)

Sugarcane (Saccharum officinalis)

Therapeutic Effects of Jupiter Plants:

Stimulating, antispasmodic, balsamic, emollient, anthelmintic, and the hepatic circulatory effect.

Plants which are Subject to Particularly the Mars

Senna (Cassia obovata)

Aleppo (Capsicum annuum) (with Saturn)

Aloe (Aloe socotrina/vera)

Pineapple (Ananas sativus)

Anemone (Anemone mexicana)

Arum (Arum maculatum)

Basil (Ocimum basilicum) (with Jupiter)
Benedict thistle (Carduus benedictus)
Barberry (Berberis vulgaris) (with Uranus)
Bloodroot (Tormentilla Brechnus) (with Sun)
Strychnine (Strychnus nux vomica)
Plantain (Plantago major) (with Sun)
Boxwood (Buxus sempervirens)
Chinese rhubarb (Rheum palmatum) (with Jupiter)
Oak (Quercus robur) (with Jupiter)
Yellow Gentian (Genista tinctoria)
Madder (Rubia tinctorum) (with Jupiter)
Daisy (Bellis perennis) (with Moon)
Honeysuckle (Lonicera caprifolium) (with Mercury)
Cursed Buttercup (Ranunculus sceleratus) (with Venus)
God's grace cabbage (Gratiola officinalis) (with Moon)
Stinging nettle (Urtica dioica) (with Pluto)
Restharrow (Ononis spinosa)
Dog Rose (Rosa canina) (with Jupiter)
Hops (Humulus lupulus)
Catnip (Nepeta cataria)
Everlasting (Helichrysum arenarium)
Pine (Pinus several species)
Small Nettle (Urtica urens) (with Pluto)
Garlic (Allium sativum)
Nodular Figwort (Scrophularia nodosa)
Cilantro (Coriandrum sativum) (with Venus)
Onion (Allium cepa)
Linseed (Linum usatissimum) (with Jupiter and Saturn)
Cochlearia Armoracia (Horseradish)

Squill (Scilla maritima) (with Saturn)

Sweet pepper (Capsicum several species)

Red bryony (Bryonia dioica)

Ruprecht herb (Geranium robertianum) (with Venus)

Sabina (Juniperus Sabina)

Sarsaparilla (Smilax utilis/Sarsaparill wurzel)

Black Radish (Raphanus sativus)

Spurge Laurel (Daphne Mezereum)

Mustard (Sinapis arvensis)

Tobacco (Nicotiana tabacum)

Hawthorn (Crataegus oxyacantha) (with Saturn)

White dead nettle (Lamium album)

Absinthe (Artemisia absinthium) (with Venus and Mercury)

Dwarf elderberry (Sambucus ebulus)

Therapeutic Effects of Mars Plants:

Aphrodisiac, stimulant, tonic, blood-forming effect on the blood vessels.

Plants which are Subject to Particularly the Mercury

Field mint (Calamintha arvensis)

Wattles (Acacia species)

Elecampane (Inula helenium)

Alraune (Mandragora officinarum) (with Saturn and the Moon)

Anise (Pimpinella anisum)

Dog's Mercury (Mercurialis perennis)

Azalea (Rhododendron spp. several species)

Valerian (Valeriana officinalis)

Mountain mint (Calamintha montana)

Bittersweet (Solanum dulcamara)

Savory (Satureja hortensis)

Strychnine (Strychnos nux vomica)

Dill (Anethum graveolens)
Wild Marjoram (Origanum vulgare)
Southernwood (Artemisia abrotanum)
Real dog tongue (Cynoglossum officinale) (with Jupiter)
Dog's Mercury (Mercurialis annua)
Endive (Cichorium endive)
Fennel (Foeniculum vulgare)
Menyanthes, bitter clover (Trifolium fibrinum)
Maidenhair (Adiantum capillus veneris)
Honeysuckle (Lonicera caprifolium)
Pellitory (Parietaria officinalis)
Oats (Avena sativa) (with Jupiter)
Hazel/Walnut (Corylus avellana)
Coltsfoot (Tussilago farfara) (with Jupiter)
Garlic Mustard (Alliaria officinalis)
Cubeb (Piper cubeba)
Caraway (Carum carvi)
Lavender (Lavandula vera) (with Jupiter and Sun)
Lily of the Valley (Convallaria majalis) (with Moon)
Marjoram (Majorana hortensis) (with sun)
Mulberry (Morus alba/Morus nigra)
Klee mice/Rabbits clover (Trifolium arvense)
Carrot (Daucus carota)
Myrtle (Myrtus communis)
Parsnip (Pastinaca sativa)
Parsley (Petroselinum hortense)
Foxglove (Digitalis purpurea) (with Venus and Saturn)
Water Germander (Teucrium scordium)
Celery (Apium graveolens)

Licorice (Glycyrrhiza glabra)

White Horehound (Marrubium vulgare)

Absinthe (Artemisia absinthium) (with Venus)

Bryony (Bryonia alba)

Therapeutic Effects of Mercurial Plants:

Retuning effects on the brain and the nervous system and regulating effects on the menstrual mechanism.

Plants which are Subject to Particularly the Moon

Oyster (Acanthus mollis)

Pale iris (Iris pallida) (with Saturn)

Watercress (Nasturtium officinale)

German iris (Iris germanica) (with Saturn)

Speedwell (Veronica officinalis)

Stonecrop (Telephium vulgare)

Florentine iris (Iris florentina) (with Saturn)

Daisy (Bellis perennis)

Turmeric (Curcuma longa)

Wallflower (Cheiranthus cheiri)

Cucumber (Cucumis sativus)

Chickweed (Stellaria media)

Periwinkle (Vinca minor)

Poppy (Papaver rhoeas) (with Saturn)

Adhesive cleaver (Galium aparine)

Small hawkweed (Hieracium pilosella)

Cabbage (Brassica oleracea)

Lettuce (Lactuca sativa)

Pumpkin (Cucurbita pepo)

Privet (Ligustrum vulgare)

Linde (Tilia spp.) (with Venus)

Saltbush/Orache (Atriplex sylvestris)

Melon tree (Carica papaya)

Vitex (Agnus castus)

Moonwort (Ruta lunaria)

Nutmeg (Myristica fragrans)

Creeping Jenny (Lysimachia nummularia)

Biting Stonecrop (Sedum acre)

Opium poppy (Papaver somniferum) (with Saturn)

Saxifrage (Saxifraga several species)

Pin Oak (Quercus palustris)

Water caltrop (Trapa natans)

Rose water (Nymphaea alba)

Willow (Salice several species)

White Lily (Lilium album)

Smock (Cardamine pratense)

Wound herb (Sedum telephium)

Hyssop (Hyssopus officinalis)

Therapeutic effect of the Moon Plants:

Alternating mind, cooling, humidity configuration; enzyme and fermentation-promoting.

Plants which are subject to particularly the Saturn

Horsetail (Equisetum arvense)

Aloe (Aloe Socotrina/Aloe Vera) (with Mars)

Alraune (Mandragora officinarum) (with Mercury and Moon)

Comfrey (Symphytum officinale) (with Jupiter)

Bittersweet (Solanum dulcamara)

Nightshade (Solanaceae) several species

Pale iris (Iris pallida) (with Moon)

Monkshood (Aconitum napellus) (with Mars)

Fenugreek (Foenum graecum)

Beech (Fagus sylvatica)

German iris (Iris germanica) (with Moon)
Ivy (Hedera helix)
Yew (Taxus baccata)
Fern (Polypodium vulgare)
Fumitory (Fumaria officinalis)
Buckthorn (Rhamnus frangula)
Box-holly (Eryngium campestre)
Sea holly (Eryngium planum)
Knapweed (Centaurea nigra)
Florentine iris (Iris Florentina) (with Moon)
Ground Elder (Aegopodium podagraria)
Barley (Hordeum vulgare)
Large-flowered mullein (Verbascum thapsiforme)
Hawkweed (Hieracium pilosella)
Hemp (Cannabis sativa) (with Neptune)
Hashish (Cannabis indica) (with Neptune)
Shepherd's purse (Capsella bursa pastoris)
Elderberry (Sambucus nigra) (with Mercury and Venus)
Elderberry sponge (Auricularia judae)
Periwinkle (Vinca minor) (with Moon)
Scots pine (Pinus silvestris)
Poppy (Papaver rhoeas) (with Moon)
Burdock (Arctium lappa) (with Venus)
Royal fern (Osmunda regalis)
Cornflower (Centaurea cvanus)
Crow (Plantago coronopus)
Onion (Allium cepa) (with Mars and Moon)
Cumin (Cuminum cyminum) (with Mercury)
Caraway (Carum carvi)
Flax (Linum usitatissimum) (with Jupiter and Mars)

Corn (Zea mays)

Sea beach thistle (Eryngium maritimum)

Squill (Scilla maritima) (with Mars)

Crested Hart's Tongue Fern (Asplenium scolopendrium/Phyllitis scolopendrium)

Golden Saxifrage (Chrysosplenium alternifolium)

Common medlar (Mespilus germanica)

Medlar Hellebore/Christmas rose (Helleborus niger)

Poplar (Populus several species) (with Jupiter and Sun)

Psyllium (Plantago ovata)

Quince (Cydonia vulgaris)

Rye (Secale cereale)

Beetroot (Beta vulgaris)

Foxglove (Digitalis purpurea) (with Mercury and Venus)

Red Chard (Beta rubra)

Solomon's Seal (Polygonatum officinale)

Amarant (Samtblume Amaranthus)

Hemlock (Conium maculatum) (with Neptune and Uranus)

Opium poppy (Papaver somniferum) (with Moon)

Blackthorn (Prunus spinosa)

Black henbane (Hyoscyamus niger) (with Jupiter and Neptune)

Senna (Senna alexandrina)

Sperber (Sorbus domestica)

Holly (Ilex aquifolium)

Pansy (Viola tricolor)

Tamarind (Tamarindus indica)

Tumble weeds (Lolium temulentum)

Belladonna (Atropa belladonna) (with Mars)

Elm (Ulmus campestris) (with Mercury)

Knotweed (Polygonum aviculare)

Chickweed (Stellaria media)

Water hemlock (Cicuta virosa)

Willow herb (Epilobium angustifolium)

Hawthorn (Crataegus oxvacantha) (with Mars)

White Hellebore (Veratrum album)

Wintergreen (Gaultheria procumbens)

Wool flower (Verbascum phlomoides)

Fern Filix mas (Aspidium filix mas)

Eggleaf twayblade (Listera ovata)

Therapeutic effects of Saturnian Plants:

Stimulating, astringent, soothing, coagulierend, mineralizing bone-forming.

Plants which are Subject to Particularly the Sun

Pimpernel (Anagallis arvensis) (with Jupiter)

Elecampane (Inula helenium)

Eyebright (Euphrasia officinalis)

Bergamot (Citrus bergamium)

Plantain (Plantago major) (with Mars)

German chamomile (Matricaria chamomilla)

Dittany (Dictamnus albus)

Marshmallow (Althaea officinalis) (with Jupiter and Venus)

Angelica (Angelica archangelica) (with Venus)

Ash (Fraxinus excelsior) (with Jupiter)

Cinquefoil (Potentilla reptans)

Yellow gentian (Gentiana lutea) (with Jupiter)

Clove tree (Syzygium aromaticum)

Clove Pink (Caryophyllus several species)

Ground ivy (Glechoma hederacea) (with Venus)

Ginger (Zingiber officinale)

St. John's Wort (Hypericum perforatum)

Calamus (Acorus calamus)
Laurel (Laurus nobilis) (with Jupiter)
Mistletoe (Viscum album) (with Jupiter and the Moon)
Blue Bedder (Echium vulgare)
Olive (Olea europaea) (with Jupiter)
Orange (Citrus aurantium)
Passion flower (Passiflora incarnata)
Pepper (Piper nigrum)
Peony (Paeonia officinalis)
Rice (Oryza satiya)
Calendula (Calendula officinalis)
Roman Chamomile (Anthemis nobilis)
Rosemary (Rosmarinus officinalis)
Celandine (Chelidonium majus) (with Jupiter)
Black mustard (Sinapis nigra)
Sunflower (Helianthus anuus)
Sundew (Drosera rotundilfolia)
Plantain (Plantago lanceolata) (with Mars)
Centaury (Centaurium Eritrea/Centaurium umbellatum)
Juniper (Juniperus communis) (with Jupiter and Mercury)
Wild Strawberry (Fragaria vesca) (with Jupiter)
Walnut (Juglans regia) (with Mercury)
Rue (Ruta graveolens)
Vine (Vitis vinifera) (with Jupiter)
White mustard (Sinapis alba)
Wild Angel (Angelica silvestris) (with Venus)
Ceylon (Cinnamonum cevlanicum)
Lemon Tree (Citrus limonum)
Lemon balm (Melissa officinalis) (with Jupiter)
Zedoary (Curcuma zedoaria)

The whole family of Labiatae is heat-and sun-related as well especially essential oils, which the volatile Sulphur (Apollo) represent.

Therapeutic effects of Solar Plants:

Toning, stimulating warm and sweaty, effect on circulation, heart, Thvmus, spleen, eyes

Plants which are Subject to Particularly the Venus

Columbine (Aquilegia vulgaris)

Apple (Pyrus malus) (with Sun)

Artichoke (Cynara scolymus)

Bearwort (Meum athamanthicum)

Mugwort (Artemisia verlotiorum) (with Mercury and Mars)

Silver Birch (Betula pendula)

Downy Birch (Betula pubescens)

Pear (Pyrus communis)

Bramble (Rubus fruticosus)

Bush bean (Phaseolus vulgaris) (with Moon)

Marshmallow (Althaea officinalis) (with Sun and Jupiter)

Verbena (Verbena officinalis) (with Mars and the Sun)

Lady's mantle (Alchemilla vulgaris)

Spring primrose (Primula officinalis) (with Sun)

Garden thyme (Thymus vulgaris) (with Sun)

Groundsel (Senecio vulgaris)

Bugelweed (Ajuga reptans)

Ground ivy (Glechoma hedera) (with Sun)

Motherwort (Leonurus cardiaca)

Elderberry (Sambucus nigra) (with Saturn and Mercury)

Ragwort (Senecio jacobaea)

Teasel (Dipsacus sativus)

Chestnut (Castanea sativa) (with Jupiter)

Catmint (Catnip Nepeta)
Chickpea (Cicer arietinum)
Small sea millet (Lithospermum minus)
Burdock (Arctium lappa)
Menthae (Mint several species)
Navelwort (Cotyledon umbilicus)
Orchis (Orchid several species)
Peach (Persica vulgaris)
Rose (Rosa damascena) (with Jupiter)
Red ox tongue (Alcanna tinctoria)
Foxglove (Digitalis purpurea) (with Mercury and Saturn)
Ruprecht (Geranium robertianum) (with Mars)
Sanicula (Sanikel europaea)
Sorrel (Rumex acetosa)
Sour Cherry (Prunus cerasus)
Sorrel (Oxalis acetosella)
Yarrow (Achillea millefolium)
Soapwort (Saponaria officinalis)
Violet (Viola odorata) (with Moon)
Wild Strawberry (Fragaria vesca) (with Sun and Jupiter)
Wheat (Triticum sativum) (with Jupiter)
Wormwood (Artemisia absinthium) (with Mercury and Mars)
Wild goldenrod (Solidago virgaurea)
Wild Thyme (Thymus serpyllum) (with Sun)

Therapeutic effects of Venusian plants:

Conversion, diuretic, antinephritic, softening, vomiting, harmonizing.

Another technique for using the planetary system of healing is the constitutional approach. This method involves a more in-depth study of the whole self, rather than just the treatment of passing symptoms and illnesses, but it offers much deeper and longer lasting true balancing and wellness. In this approach, the birth information of the patient is examined, and a planetary rulership is determined for each of three levels of being, corresponding to the classic alchemical Salt, Mercury, and Sulfur. The concept behind this is that at the time of birth, the planetary energies created a sort of "snapshot" of that moment within each of us, stamping their influences and energies at each level of being. The rulership of each of these levels determines all types of qualities, such as strengths, weaknesses, disease and health tendencies, and affinities for certain methods of treatment.

Since disease tendencies are often found within the constitutional picture, working with the constitution is often very effective in treating illness in a targeted, personal way. But more importantly, planetary constitutional support works to support the native vital energy at the deepest level, helping to avoid disease entirely by keeping proper balance. The idea behind this is a simple but profound one, if you stay well, you will not become sick. This technique is a truly holistic one, considering and working with the whole self of both the plant and patient.

Once health and balance are achieved, or in an already healthy person, a more aggressive approach of self-improvement can be undertaken. The planetary energies can be deliberately introduced in varying proportions to produce certain effects in the body, mind, or spiritual level of a person. For example, someone who does not have serious self-esteem problems or related disorders, but who would like to become more confident or charismatic can work with a Sun-ruled Spagyric to introduce more of that energy, or, rather than just accenting one specific quality, each planetary influence can be explored and worked with in turn to create an energetic and spiritual balance with all influences both without and within. This method of working, when integrated into the individual's own spiritual work, is a powerful technique for personal improvement.

In-depth discussion on the various methods of using planetary healing, and analysis of specific pathways in which the individual planets interact within the body, and how these interactions of support and opposition can be used as tools for healing are given below. We will review how to discover your personal planetary constitution, and how to target spagyrics to both the level and ruling planet of each of the three parts of that constitution.

Healing at all Three Levels

We have discussed some basic ideas of spagyric and alchemical work, and how these ideas can be applied as part of a healing system. We also explained the role that the seven classical planetary energies and archetypes play in this system, and examined the qualities and energies of each of the planets. We introduced some methods for working on a practical level with these energies, from the simple work with a planet ruling an organ to be worked on, to the more complex system of constitutional healing. Finally, we mentioned some approaches to integrating the planetary energies into the self at the higher levels of being in order to bring about spiritual growth.

To begin explaining these ideas and techniques in-depth, we will start with the simplest approach, which uses planetary sympathy and antipathy to bring balance to the being.

In this approach, the starting point is the planetary energies and their rulerships and attributes, as explained in the second article. Each planet rules organs and organ systems, as well as herbs and the healing effects they manifest. These rulerships are called sympathies, and working with sympathy is the simplest way to integrate medicinal alchemy into healing work.

This work of sympathy is a way of working with the chain of influence that begins at each planet, arriving on earth and affecting its inhabitants. Each planet's energy has an affinity for some types of healing effects over others, and each herb manifests more of one planet's energy than others. By starting with a plant ruled by a certain planet, and then working on that plant alchemically and spagyrically to focus and magnify that energetic rulership, another link in that chain is created. The final link is made when the spagyric medicine is chosen and taken to support the imbalanced organ, according to its rulership. By supplying that organ with the planetary energy which is at the core of its function and being, a greater balance is achieved, and a more harmonious constellation of inner energies is created, mirroring the outer one of the universe.

This sympathetical support approach is a simple and direct way of achieving balance, and is analogous to taking vitamins, which do not usually have a direct effect upon disease, but help the overall functioning of the body in its own efforts to heal. A more direct approach, which is targeted at specific ailments, is working with antipathy.

All philosophies and spiritual systems acknowledge the existence of pairs of opposites: yin/yang, male/female, etc. The planets, too, follow this pattern, and their actions of opposing or modifying each other can be used as healing tools.

As stated before, diseases are ruled by the planetary energies, both according to the organs affected and to the qualities, actions, and results of the disease. Some diseases are hot or cold, or wet or dry, some have to do with building up and some with degeneration. Looking beyond the simple organ rulership to examine other potential energies involved in the imbalance is like doing surgery with a scalpel instead of a machete. The following rough outline of some of these effects can be used as a start to this work.

Moon

The Moon rules any diseases which are cold or wet in nature. It should be noted that, in this system, we think of temperatures both in literal terms and as effects or actions, in much the same way as Ayurvedic or Chinese medicine do. Thus, "cold" can mean literally cold, as in hypothermia, or it can mean stagnant, not moving, inactive, or dull. Some examples of that type of cold would be edema or water retention, or sprains and injuries which are swollen and not clearing up. These examples also show the wet aspect of lunar problems. Poor circulation is a cold ailment both literally and energetically, and sinus congestion is another example of a wet imbalance.

For antipathy, the Moon's influence is most used against the Sun's imbalances. A good example of this is sunburn, an obvious disorder from the sun, which is helped by the cooling and moisturizing effects of the lunar herbs aloe and cucumber.

Secondly, the soothing, relaxing effects of moon herbs can be helpful in problems caused by the aggressive, stimulating effects of Mars, another hot planet. An example would be the common use of Passionflower in cases of stress or hypertension.

Mars

Mars rules any diseases which are hot, active, or related to stimulation. Fever is the most common example, along with swellings which are hot, as opposed to the stagnant swelling of the Moon. Rashes and irritations are also ruled by Mars, as are any illnesses caused by stress or aggression, such as ulcers or hypertension.

The primary opposite of Mars is Venus. This opposition is best illustrated by the interplay of organs and effects occurring in venereal disease. Ruled by Venus (hence the name) and manifesting on her organ of the skin, it also affects the sexual organs of Mars. Mars rules lust and sexuality, whereas Venus rules the higher love which transcends the physical. When there is overindulgence in the Mars level of love, its opposite Venus becomes imbalanced. Both planets are useful in treatment, Venus for skin-toning effects, and Mars to support the immune system.

The other energetic interaction for Mars is with the Moon, as described above from the Moon's perspective. The wet, congested, boggy or poorly healing conditions ruled by the Moon are often helped by Mars's action of stimulation, heating, and movement. Mars can also be used to give more force to any other planets' influence.

Mercury

The swift messenger and go-between, Mercury rules any imbalances of balance that is, any problem arising from lack of adaptability or preponderance of one energy over another. Mercury does not have a clear opposite as the other planets do, rather, it contains within itself a complete set of sympathies and antipathies. This coherence gives Mercury a strong intelligence towards balancing and adaptation, helpful in cases of lack or excess. Mercury herbs are most often marked by this paradoxical ability; as non-specific balancers and adaptogens, they are the great helpers of the plant world. Another important manifestation of Mercury is the adaptation of Mercury herbs as helpers in formulas. In

Chinese medicine, for example, Licorice is used for its specific effects, but also to make formulas more palatable, and to lessen side effects from other herbs and focus and direct their action.

Jupiter

Jupiter rules expansion, growth, and the anabolic processes of the body. Jupiter also rules judgement, both in the mental sense and in the sense of the organs' and cells' reactions to processes and situations. Consciously overeating is an example of a Jupiter imbalance, but being overweight even with a sensible diet is Jupiter as well. In that last, more subtle case, the imbalance of Jupiter is seen at the cellular level, where calories and food are stored as unnecessary fat instead of burned off, a sort of poor judgement of the metabolism. Any building up or increase of tissues which is unhealthy, then, would be Jupiter, from the overeating example to tumor growth.

Jupiter's opposite is Saturn, and Jupiter's open, expansive qualities can be used to counteract the cold, dry contraction of Saturn. A good example of this would be any type of stone or calcium buildup, as in the kidneys, which would be ruled by Saturn's hard mineralizing influence. Many herbs which help break up and remove stones are ruled by Jupiter, and act by stimulating bile in Jupiter's organ, the liver.

Jupiter can also be used where tissue growth and weight buildup are wanted, as in recovering from a long illness (chronic, slow or long-term and wasting diseases are ruled by Saturn) or in eating disorders.

Venus

Venus rules the kidneys, skin, and the heart chakra. Venus also rules beauty, the arts, refinement, and true love of a high, spiritual nature. Venus's influence is seen in herbs which are astringent and toning to the skin, cleansing in a mild, non-purgative way, and, on a spiritual level, in herbs which promote affection and closeness, or are aphrodisiac.

As stated above, Venus is opposite to Mars, who focuses on many of the same relationship issues, but in a more gross physical way. Venus can be used to temper this influence and bring more spiritual aspects to relationships. Venus's beneficial influence on the skin is most often useful in cases of Mars ruled rashes, irritations, and infections, as seen in the common use of Venus-ruled Witch Hazel to treat scrapes, rashes, and acne. Venus can also be used where toning and astringency are needed, but the overly shrinking or drying action of Saturn would not be wanted.

Saturn

Saturn's influence is cold, shrinking, drying, and stabilizing. Saturn rules the mineral and structural tissues of the bones and teeth, and mineral buildup in general, especially calcium, as discussed above. This mineralizing effect can be useful in cases of broken bones or poorly healing injuries.

Saturn's shrinking, drying influence can almost be like squeezing a sponge, draining the tissues of the body. This can be used to tone the tissues and detoxify to remove Jupiter's unwanted weight, and to help clear up injuries and swellings when Mars's action could be too heating or stimulating. Yerba Mansa is a southwestern herb of Saturn, much used in cases of arthritis, an ailment of the bones and toxic buildup in the joints, causing inflammation which would be further aggravated if Mars was used to stimulate clearing of the joints. This example is one of both sympathy and antipathy, of organ support (bones) and disease opposition (shrinking of inflamed joints).

Sun

The Sun is warming and stimulating, but not in as tense a way as Mars. Mars stimulates and clears influences, purging them from the body, whereas the Sun relaxes and opens, moving energy around the body. This is why, for poor circulation and the associated coldness of the extremities, Mars may seem initially to be the best warming choice, but actually Sun is preferred. Mars herbs, such as cayenne, do initially stimulate circulation and warm the body, but this warming influence extends past the boundary of the skin, outwards through sweat, which eventually has a cooling effect. The Sun, too, stimulates warmth, as with Ginger, but this warmth is circulated through the body, not pushed and purged outwards, and so is more effective.

It is interesting to note that many solar herbs are considered uplifting, cheering and anti-depressant, in much the same way as the Sun itself, coming out from behind clouds. The Sun's opposite, the Moon, rules the night, and rules many "dark" disorders such as depression. St. John's Wort is a suddenly popular example of using the Sun in antipathy to the Moon, and is often helpful in Seasonal Affective Disorder, which has many lunar aspects: a cyclical nature, emotional upset, and arising from lack of sunlight.

This list is in not comprehensive, but it should be a good start to supplementing simple organ support, according to the rulerships described in the previous article, with a more targeted and directed attack on ailments and imbalances.

The second level of healing work is the Alchemical Constitutional system which we developed. This system works with the classic alchemical levels of being- Salt, Mercury, and Sulfur. These three aspects of being are considered the energetic building blocks of all natural things, and humans are no exception.

Our innovative system of constitutional medicine works with the three levels as a diagnostic tool, in which each of us has a specific planetary rulership on each of these levels, determined by examining the date and time of birth. At that moment, a sort of energetic snapshot was taken and imprinted on each of us, in much the same way as a traditional astrological chart is considered a picture of your being. While the traditional astrological chart is a picture of various influences from all aspects of life, such as love, career, and so on, the constitutional rulership is specific to your health and wellness, and to ways of maintaining balance and health in an individualized way.

The first level of the constitution is the Salt level, corresponding to the physical body and its attributes. Salt is the lowest and most dense level, the level of solidity, the body and the physical being. In Alchemical healing, the Salt level corresponds to the physical body of a person, different for each of us, and reflecting in a material way the more ethereal aspects of our selves. This is not always the level of the root causes of illness, but it is often the level at which symptoms manifest. The planetary rulership of the Salt level gives insights into the physical qualities, weaknesses, and disease tendencies for each of us.

The Salt level moves on a cycle of planetary influences in 3 hour 26 minute intervals, the result of dividing a 24-hour day into seven periods. This cycle, shown in this chart, is seen in Vedic astrology.

Planetary Rulerships of the Salt and Mercury Levels

Daily Rulership:	*Sunday*	*Monday*	*Tuesday*	*Wednesday*	*Thursday*	*Friday*	*Saturday*
Mercury	*Sun*	*Moon*	*Mars*	*Mercury*	*Jupiter*	*Venus*	*Saturn*
Hourly Rulerships:							
Salt							
12:00 am–3:25 am	Mars	Mercury	Jupiter	Venus	Saturn	Sun	Moon
3:25 am–6:51 am	Sun	Moon	Mars	Mercury	Jupiter	Venus	Saturn
6:51 am–10:17 am	Venus	Saturn	Sun	Moon	Mars	Mercury	Jupiter
10:17 am–1:42 pm	Mercury	Jupiter	Venus	Saturn	Sun	Moon	Mars
1:42 pm–5:08 pm	Moon	Mars	Mercury	Jupiter	Venus	Saturn	Sun
5:08 pm–8:34 pm	Saturn	Sun	Moon	Mars	Mercury	Jupiter	Venus
8:34 pm–12:00 am	Jupiter	Venus	Saturn	Sun	Moon	Mars	Mercury

The interval from 3:25-6:51 am, the pre-dawn and dawn cycle, is the interval during which the life force, or Prana, is the strongest, and is ruled by the planet which rules that day. The successive intervals repeat in a cycle in the following order: Saturn, Jupiter, Mars, Sun, Venus, Mercury, and Moon. This is also the order of planetary influence in the descent of matter into creation, according to Qabala.

To work medicinally at this level, the hour and day of birth of the patient must be found. Then, the chart is consulted to determine the planetary rulership for the time interval during which the patient was born.

In the spagyric work with plants, the Salt resides in the mineral components of the plant and the hard structural tissues. Since alchemically all things contain the same three levels of being, to determine a plant spagyric to the Salt level of being in humans, the Salt level of the plant would be included in the tincture. This is done by making a simple tincture, at a fairly unrefined level, and adding the ash of the plant body, which is its Salt-level attribute and gives its energies body and physical being. A simple spagyric prepared this way, using a plant under the same planetary rulership as the Salt level of the person, would be used to support the physical level of being.

Mercury is the middle level of being. This is the level of fluidity, and is the spirit or life essence animating a being. The Mercury level is the mediator between the etheric, planetary energies above and the physical constellation of the body, as well as the mediator between the other two levels of being. Because of this, the Mercury level is often an effective entry point to work on imbalances, as it has the most contact with the other levels of self.

The planetary ruler of the Mercury level is the quality for which you have the most need throughout life, and determines your healthy qualities and strengths. It is also the level of imbalances from an emotional or mental cause, even if they have progressed enough to manifest physically, and the level to use to boost overall vitality and energy.

The Mercury-level rulership is determined by the day of birth, according to the common, traditional planetary daily rulership-Monday is Moon, Tuesday is Mars, Wednesday is Mercury, Thursday is Jupiter, Friday is Venus, Saturday is Saturn, and Sunday is Sun. The weekday of birth for any date can be found by using a perpetual calendar or consulting an ephemeris.

In the plant kingdom, the Mercury resides in the alcohol, which is the carrier of the life force. Using a highly concentrated and purified alcohol, and refining the plant ashes to become a pure salt, determines a spagyric to the Mercury level. Using the Mercury level of spagyric for the proper planetary rulership affects and balances the astral, mental, and emotional aspects of being, as well as boosting overall life force and vitality.

The highest level of being is Sulfur, the most subtle and etheric aspect of the self. The Sulfur is the soul, which brings the intelligence to the body, and is the inner, eternal form. From a healing perspective, the Sulfur level deals with all forms of predisposition towards or away from imbalances and diseases, including influences such as genetic tendencies, karma, or predestination, as well as diseases which recur frequently, or are deeply ingrained.

The Sulfur level is also the spiritual level of being, and the level of the soul and its accumulation of past knowledge and experience. This level is often the most difficult to treat, as it is so subtle, but the results of great spiritual imbalance can be very destructive in all areas of life, and the rewards of a balanced and meaningful spiritual life are now acknowledged by even mainstream medical researchers.

To determine the planetary ruler of this part of the constitution, the time of birth is again examined, but with a different chart, from the work of German Occult practitioner Heinrich Cornelius Agrippa von Nettesheim. This chart changes each hour beginning at sunrise.

Planetary Rulerships of the Sulfur Level

Hour	*Sun.*	*Mon.*	*Tue.*	*Wed.*	*Thur.*	*Fri.*	*Sat.*
1st	Sun	Moon	Mars	Mercury	Jupiter	Venus	Saturn
2nd	Venus	Saturn	Sun	Moon	Mars	Mercury	Jupiter
3rd	Mercury	Jupiter	Venus	Saturn	Sun	Moon	Mars
4th	Moon	Mars	Mercury	Jupiter	Venus	Saturn	Sun
5th	Saturn	Sun	Moon	Mars	Mercury	Jupiter	Venus
6th	Jupiter	Venus	Saturn	Sun	Moon	Mars	Mercury
7th	Mars	Mercury	Jupiter	Venus	Saturn	Sun	Moon
8th	Sun	Moon	Mars	Mercury	Jupiter	Venus	Saturn
9th	Venus	Saturn	Sun	Moon	Mars	Mercury	Jupiter
10th	Mercury	Jupiter	Venus	Saturn	Sun	Moon	Mars
11th	Moon	Mars	Mercury	Jupiter	Venus	Saturn	Sun
12th	Saturn	Sun	Moon	Mars	Mercury	Jupiter	Venus
13th	Jupiter	Venus	Saturn	Sun	Moon	Mars	Mercury
14th	Mars	Mercury	Jupiter	Venus	Saturn	Sun	Moon
15th	Sun	Moon	Mars	Mercury	Jupiter	Venus	Saturn
16th	Venus	Saturn	Sun	Moon	Mars	Mercury	Jupiter
17th	Mercury	Jupiter	Venus	Saturn	Sun	Moon	Mars
18th	Moon	Mars	Mercury	Jupiter	Venus	Saturn	Sun
19th	Saturn	Sun	Moon	Mars	Mercury	Jupiter	Venus
20th	Jupiter	Venus	Saturn	Sun	Moon	Mars	Mercury
21st	Mars	Mercury	Jupiter	Venus	Saturn	Sun	Moon
22nd	Sun	Moon	Mars	Mercury	Jupiter	Venus	Saturn
23rd	Venus	Saturn	Sun	Moon	Mars	Mercury	Jupiter
24th	Mercury	Jupiter	Venus	Saturn	Sun	Moon	Mars

To use this chart, it is necessary to know the day and time of the patient's birth, as before, and also to know the time of sunrise on that day, in the place where the patient was born. The time of sunrise begins the first hour in the "Hour" column. To find the patient's planetary ruler, go down the hour column until you reach the one-hour period after sunrise during which the patient was born. Then, go across the columns until you are in the column of the day on which the patient was born. There you will find the planetary ruler of the Sulfur level.

Example: a patient born at 2:30 pm on a Tuesday, on which the sun rose at 5:45 am. That day, 5:45-6:45 am was the first hour, 6:45-7:45 am was the second hour, etc. Therefore, the birth at 2:30 pm occurred during the ninth hour of that day, which, on Tuesday, is ruled by the Sun.

In the plant kingdom, the Sulfur resides in the essential oils. Essential oils are the soul of a plant, as well as being the carrier of scent, the most etheric aspect of plants. To create a spagyric which is directed at the soul body, all aspects of the extract should be as refined as possible, so that they become more spiritual or etheric than physical, and the essential oils should be the main focus of the extraction process.

Working at this level balances the planetary energies according to their pure energetic qualities, which may or may not affect physical health. The work with the Sulfur level supports the soul level of being, by entering vibrationally at the soul level and adjusting it to a higher state of being. When this higher state of being is achieved, it is as if the lower vibrations of disease cannot reach you, and the state of balanced health is much easier to maintain.

More importantly, though, the Sulfur-level work begins the work of personal spiritual growth and development, bringing the planetary balance to the internal subtle qualities, and enabling more powerful and successful magickal or spiritual work with the planetary archetypes. By working to strengthen and fortify yourself at this level, a more refined and strong spiritual body is created, which can then go on to the advancement, development, and personal perfection that is the aim of alchemy.

Ens:

Ens is a word created by Paracelsus to describe a vital force or energy which is within all natural things. Our organs and body systems have individual Ens, and when the Ens is strong, health and balance are present. Diseases also have Ens, and can overcome the healthy Ens of the body, but fortunately, plants also carry the Ens, in a form which is healing and vitalizing to us. Count Cesare Mattei termed this energy as Od Force.

Energetic Medicine and Vitalism

Beginning in the last half of the 1700's, a new current of thought and system of working began to appear in medical practice. This new way of looking at health, disease, the body, and medicine was characterized by a focus on the inner energetic or vital aspect of the body, organs, and plants, and this system eventually became known as Vitalism.

The study of Vitalism became integrated into many of the popular treatment modalities of the time, including Homeopathic and Spagyric medicine.

Drawing on many ancient sources, particularly Hippocrates and Paracelsus, the Vitalist doctors and writers of the time sought to heal the body not by opposing or suppressing the symptoms and manifestations of disease, but by supporting the body's own innate ability to heal itself.

Every illness creates an imbalance, and what conventional medicine often defines as the illness is often a strong reaction in one direction produced by the body in an effort to heal itself. Thus, body functions such as fever, coughing, or runny nose should not be suppressed, but seen as indications of an imbalance which should be acted on at the deeper level of its origin.

None of this is new to modern holistic healers; the idea that "the natural healing force within us is the greatest force in getting well", as Hippocrates put it, is well integrated into all forms of holistic health care. What may be less familiar to most healers, though, is how these ideas appear in alchemy and Spagyrics, and particularly our work.

Plants, too, have an inner vital force, and this vitalism acts to protect the plant by modifying the physical qualities and functions of the plant, in much the same way as a human body might create a fever to deal with infection. In Alchemy, this ability to respond to protect the inner life is called "intelligence", and it appears in the myriad ways in which plants survive.

Because of the natural affinity that plants and animals have, many of the physical qualities created by this intelligence are useful in healing. A plant like Osha, for example, grows in places that are cold, wet, and shaded, an environment which is perfect for mold and rot. Osha responds by creating some of the strongest antifungal and antibacterial substances in the plant kingdom, substances which are so strong that it is almost impossible to get Osha roots to rot. When properly extracted, these substances, and the protective intelligence behind them, become one of the best natural medicines for infection in the body, especially the moist, cool tissues of the lungs.

Proper extraction is the key here, and this is where the importance of alchemy and Spagyrics is shown. Many healing systems work with the tendencies of plants, on both physical and energetic levels, but most of these healing systems isolate only one aspect of a plant's action. Conventional herbalism is increasingly focused on the chemical constituents of the plant and on isolating what is defined as the "active" constituent. Homeopathy, by using rounds of succussion and dilution, leaves very little or none of the plant's chemicals in the final medicine, focusing instead on the pure energetic qualities of the remedy. Both of these approaches, however natural and useful they may be, are a type of isolation, in which only one of the plant's reactions or abilities is used, and on only one level.

By concentrating and purifying the physical and chemical aspects of the plant, while carefully working to protect and magnify the original intelligence that creates the healing qualities, Spagyric processing follows a path of synthesis. Both chemistry and intelligence are purified and taken to their highest possible level in laboratory operations that are a continuation of the plant's own growth process.

The results are extracts which perfectly fit the Vitalist work handed down since ancient times, which should be at the root of healing today. The concentrated chemical constituents work to balance and heal the physical body, while the purified and focused vital intelligence directs their action and synergistically transfers the plant's life force to the vital energy of the patient. This two-fold action naturally supports the body's specific and symptomatic efforts to re-balance itself as well as bringing the whole being into a higher state of balance above the level of the original illness.

The best and most simple way to work within this system is to follow a two-part approach. First, any specific or short-term ailments or imbalances should be worked on and rebalanced using our Spagyric Essences or Essences Plus. This level of Spagyric is created to operate mainly on the physical being, and can be used to support the body's natural efforts to deal with an illness, or to oppose any overactive or harmful reactions the body may have, such as dangerously high fevers, excessive coughing, etc.

Although the Essence-level Spagyrics are created to work on the physical level, all levels of being are considered and worked with in their creation, so that they carry the plant's vital force and act with much greater efficiency, more balance, and fewer unwanted effects than conventionally-made medicines.

After any short-term, acute, or passing imbalances are worked out, the next phase of work is to go on to achieve long-term wellness, vitality, and longevity. For this work, strengths, weaknesses, disease histories and tendencies should all be considered, and a plan of health goals and needs should be worked out. Then, a system of health improvement similar to the Ayurvedic Rasayana work is undertaken, with the goal of preservation, rejuvenation, and longevity.

The Spagyric for this phase of work is the Spiritualized Essence, described in the next article.

Quintessential Healing

One of the most important ideas of Alchemy and Spagyrics is expressed in the originally alchemical word *quintessence*. In ordinary parlance, quintessence has come to mean the best or purest part or expression of a thing, or the part without which the whole could not exist.

The alchemical origins of this word have a deeper meaning, hinted at in the two root words, *quinta* or fifth, and *essentia* or essence. The fifth essence referred to is the vital realm of etheric and subtle qualities, above the four lower essences or elements of earth, water, air, and fire. This quintessence is both above the four lower ones and a product of them, as it is in the purification of physical that it originates. It is described as "the quality of substances separated by Art from the body" and the "Mysterium, exalted to the purity of ethereal nature, and the highest virtues".

Just as the physical actions of a plant have a deeper root in the intelligence, the intelligence comes from a deeper level of the plant's being, its true inner life force. The plant, then, is made up of three layers of being: the deepest life force, the intelligence which it creates around itself as a protection, and the sphere of action and physical qualities which are the instruments of the intelligence.

There is an affinity between plants and people, and the intelligence shown by a plant's qualities is mirrored in the intelligence of the human body and its actions. The wide variety of medicinal plants gives what seems to be an endless number of healing effects, but if we once again go back to the root intelligence, the types of herbal action fall into only a few categories, and most relate to organs of the body. In our work, the body's organs and the plants which affect them are organized according to the alchemical archetypes of the planets.

These therapeutic actions and organ affinities are preserved in our work, but our processing is unique in that it refines the Spiritualized Essence to a level of overall support of the vital energy of whole organs and organ systems, rather than just one of the organ's actions or functions.

By focusing our processing on the plant's intelligence and life force that are the heart of its healing properties, the natural affinity that plants have for humans becomes a synergy, and the body's ability to truly adapt instead of merely reacting is supported. This support of true wellness enables the body to stop the peaks-and-valleys syndrome that is so common in illness and healing, which leaves drained even when an illness has been successfully fought off.

To work with the Spiritualized Essences in healing practice, any specific imbalances, illnesses, or symptoms should first be eliminated using Essences. Then, more long-term health plans should be worked out for the patient. This lifetime approach should consider factors such as past illnesses and any continuing weaknesses, family history, and lifestyle.

After evaluating these variables, areas of the patient's life and health will be found which need more support than others. These areas, which generally correspond to organs or organ systems, can then be supported with a Spiritualized Essence.

Such an ongoing health plan should have as its goal the preservation of functional life, not just life span, and the maintenance of perfect health on all levels of being.

This state of perfect health is the Quintessence of the body's abilities, a state of balance between all physical elements and subtle levels of being. This condition is created from the harmony between all of the aspects of our being, but is also more than this, it is the higher essence of self sought by the alchemists and achieved through their Quintessential medicines.

Improvements in our Three-Level System

Paracelsus taught that all natural things are made up of three levels of being:

Salt/ Body, Mercury/Spirit, and Sulfur/Soul.

He also stressed the importance of targeting illness with specific medicines which have been created to operate on the level of disease origin, not just its symptoms. Following this, we have created three levels of Spagyric- the Tincture, the Essence, and the Magistery.

The ashes of a plant add some components over an ordinary filtered tincture, but even the word Spagyric, meaning separate and recombine, suggests that more is possible than just burning plant matter. Philosophically, Alchemy considers ashes and charcoals to be "caput mortem", or waste products, and ancient texts never recommend that they be included in extracts.

Our process of the purification of the plant matter only starts with ashes, the end results are crystalline salts with no impurities, which contain alkaloids and minerals in Oligo form, constituents which are not metabolized or accessible from ashes. This further work means that not only is our overall product Spagyric in the true sense of the word, but that each component of the final medicine has been individually processed in a Spagyric way.

Energies, too, should be considered as part of the Spagyric process, and their purification and elevation, while more subtle and difficult, is just as important if the desired result is to be more than just physical medicine.

Paracelsus considered the etheric energies of the body and plants to be another important factor in directing healing efforts, and he used the planetary archetypes to understand, describe, and implement this extra level of healing. We work according to planetary cycles and rulerships, and perform all operations according to this timing, so that the inner nature of the plant can be magnified and its intelligence and life force protected.

This development also represents a step up of our entire system of Constitutional Healing, an evolution of our system to keep pace with the evolution and growing awareness of people today.

The Three Level Constitution

Salt

The level of the Body and physical symptoms, treated with the Spagyric Essence. The Essence is produced through two separate extractions, one by alcohol and one by water. This dual-extraction method ensures that the maximum possible amount of the plant's physical level is represented in the final Spagyric. After these extractions are done, the plant body is purified, not just to an ash, but to a white or clear crystalline salt. The Essences are more suited for working on the physical level and its greater variation of imbalances and needs.

Mercury

The level of the Spirit, life force, and vitality, accessed through the Spiritualized Essence. The plant is extracted in one long, intensive process, and the remaining plant matter is made into a salt in much the same way as in the Essence-level work.

All of the work on the Spiritualized Essences, however, takes place with much more refined ingredients and processing than the lower-level Essences. The alcohol is a higher percentage and more refined quality, the salts are Spagyrically revived, energized, and made into living salts, the overall extract is more concentrated, and the Spagyric growth cycle is longer, more active, and more complex. This processing magnifies the plant's intelligence and life force, and supports the body's adaptations and maintenance of real wellness. This adaptive quality is the primary function of the Mercury level, and the Spiritualized Essences are a perfect interface between the body's higher and lower levels.

Spiritualized Essences may be used to balance and increase vitality over a long period of time. This proactive approach of maintaining true health, beyond just the absence of disease, is similar to the Ayurvedic work of Rasayana, or rejuvenation therapy.

Sulfur

The level of the Soul and eternal qualities, supported by the Magistery. The Magistery contains every possible constituent of the plant, separated, purified, and recombined. This processing, which takes a year to complete, includes five distillations and the extraction of three different salts and two essential oils.

The Magistery supports the whole being at the highest level, the level of past causes and deeply ingrained imbalances, or imbalances from subtle or spiritual causes. The Magistery is also used to work with the higher etheric qualities of plants as part of a spiritual path of balancing and growth. Since this level is archetypal and not specific, there are eight Magisteries only, one for each planet plus Earth.

Healing the Subtle Levels

The core tenet of Paracelsus work and our own is that all natural beings exist at levels other than the obvious physical, and that all levels of being must be healed for true wellness to exist. But, since these other layers of self are so subtle, how do we begin to understand and work with them?

To us, Paracelsus's great gift has been his transmutation of the complex and often mystifying teachings of alchemy into a practical and efficient healing system. In his work, he describes three levels of being, familiar to many who work with us.

Salt is the physical level, the body and all of its functions and activities, the usual realm of conventional medicine. Most symptoms will eventually manifest at this level, although not all imbalances originate here.

The Mercury level encompasses the mind, thought, and emotions, as well as general life force or vitality. Although less apparent than the Salt level, it is easy to see the results of a Mercury level imbalance in such emotional or mentally caused disorders as ulcers or depression. A general lack of vitality and the energy to be well is also easily understood by most healers, and supporting vitality at this level is often the focus of Rasayana or Qi balancing.

Sulfur is the most subtle level of being, and often the most difficult to diagnose and treat. At the Sulfur level resides the Soul, or eternal aspect of each of us. Alchemically, the Sulfur level of all natural things is the blueprint of each being's eventual self, and the path each being will follow to realize that potential. The Sulfur level is also all types of inheritance or passed-on traits, whether from our own Karmic state or from our ancestor's genetics.

Whether as potential and path, or inherited traits, it is simpler to first understand the Sulfur level's role in plants. Alchemically, Sulfur resides in the essential oils, which are very often the source of the chemicals developed by a plant's ancestors to survive in certain conditions. The condensed genetic inheritance contained in a Rosemary seed is the blueprint for the plant it will become, giving it the ability to produce resins which will protect it from drying out in the harsh sun of its native climate. It also inherits other active chemicals, to protect it from rot, insects, or other influences encountered by past members of its kind.

After this package of inherited traits becomes a new plant, this same group of chemicals, frequently contained in the essential oils, becomes the route through which the plant will interact with its environment- its blueprint of action. These chemicals also act on us if we ingest them, and the essential oils can be the most efficient and archetypal way to let them act on us.

In people, the Sulfur level is much the same, although perhaps more complex to understand because of our greater potential for action in life. It still, however, represents the blueprint of our potential and the tools we have been given to build with. Besides genetic traits and constitutional makeup, this can also be Karmic or very entrenched imbalances, or any condition which we must always be bound by.

In a more positive light, the Sulfur level also governs our spiritual self, since it is the most subtle level and most in contact with the divine or eternal realm. An excellent example of this level's role in health is found in recent studies indicating that individuals with fulfilling spiritual lives, regardless of denomination or creed, become ill much less often and heal more quickly than those who are not as spiritually inclined.

Since alchemically there is a correlation between the three levels of being across the kingdoms of mineral, vegetable, and animal, an extract can be created from one kingdom to target the same level in another. In our Magisteries, the Spagyric extraction process is very refined and subtle, and emphasizes the essential oils of the plant used, targeting the refined and subtle Sulfur level in the eventual healing use. Magisteries are the fullest expression of all of the plant's constituents and qualities, concentrated and elevated from their raw state but still represented in their full natural spectrum and proportions.

The Magisteries can be used in healing whenever the Sulfur level is involved, whether from deeply entrenched or inherited imbalances, spiritual needs, or when the constitutional rulership of the Sulfur level indicates imbalance. They can also be of great help in an active spiritual path, as a form of immersion into any or all of the archetypal planetary energies for greater inner balance.

Primary Relationships between Planets, Metals, Days, Cardinal Sins & Virtues and Parts of the Body

The below table will help readers to find the various inter-relationships, when working with the alchemical manifestations on both, the transcendental and physical planes. Remember that each metallic substance has a spiritual counterpart manifesting at the same time, according to the law of duality. Alchemical remedies are therefore of either like or contrary nature, attracting or repulsing respectively at specific times either beneficial or inimical.

Planet	Metal	Day	Cardinal Sin	Cardinal Virtue	Part of Body
Sun	Gold	Sunday	Pride	Humility	Heart
Moon	Silver	Monday	Lust of Flesh	Substantiality	Brain
Mars	Iron	Tuesday	Anger	Meekness	Gall
Mercury	Quicksilver	Wednesday	Envy	Benevolence	Liver
Jupiter	Tin	Thursday	Cunning	Wisdom	Lungs
Venus	Copper	Friday	Lewdness	Chastity	Regen. Orgs
Saturn	Lead	Saturday	Avarice	Charity	Spleen

The Sun represents the Alchemical Element Sulphur. The Planet Mercury represents the Alchemical Element Mercury. The ruling planet of the metal (for instance, Moon for Silver) represents the Alchemical Element Salt.

Sulphur, Salt and Mercury are in all substances. Some contain more of the one, than the other, thus making possible the different manifestations of matter.

"The Roman Catholic church recognized the seven capital virtues as opposites to the Seven Capital Sins or the Seven Deadly Sins. According to Dante's The Divine Comedy the sins have an order of greatness, and the virtues a respective order of greatness as well. This order is shown below from the lowest to the highest."

Sin	Virtue
Lust (excessive sexual appetites)	Chastity (purity)
Gluttony (over-indulgence)	Temperance (self-restraint)
Greed (avarice)	Charity (giving)
Sloth (laziness/idleness)	Diligence (zeal/integrity/ Labor)
Wrath (anger)	Forgiveness (composure)
Envy (jealousy)	Kindness (admiration)
Pride (vanity)	Humility (humbleness)

Lust- An insatiable need for sex or things of a sexual nature. This includes thoughts, desires, and actions. If this need is unfed, it can lead to masturbation, rape, and even beastiality. Lust is fed by any of the aforementioned means or viewing pornography.

Gluttony- Over indulgences of anything to the extreme, usually food or drink. Alcoholism, drug abuse, etc. are considered as part of Gluttony.

Greed- Greed is the need for material possessions or material wealth. If this need is unfed, a Greedy person may even resort to hoarding their goods, theft, robbery, or obtaining any material possessions by means of trickery, violence, deception, or manipulation. Greedy people usually are easy to bribe, or will take any bet or do anything for a dollar.

Sloth- Sadness, depression, or the inability to feel joy. Sloth is often confused with Gluttony, though I don't know why. Those who suffer from depression to an extreme usually have thoughts of or plans for suicide. Many times, Sloth can lead to another sin: Wrath. Those who have lost or lack love, usually fall into a deep state of Sloth.

Wrath- Extreme anger, rage, hatred, or a need for vengeance or revenge. People who suffer with Wrath issues will often resort to taking the law in their own hands if they feel the justice system has failed them. To feed the need of Wrath, they may even turn to physical abuse of themself or others, murder, or even genocide. Wrath usually is a need to do harm to others. Dante described Wrath as "*love of justice perverted to revenge and spite.*"

Envy- The need to have better or be better than others. The need to have the goods of others. Wanting what others have for yourself. Many times, someone with extreme Envious needs may turn to voyeurism to feed the need to see what others have that the envious want.

Pride- Once considered a need to be the most beautiful, Pride can also mean a need for public acceptance in all acts. Pride can also be a need to be more important than others. Those who suffer with Pride issues, usually fail to give due complements to others, but instead fish for complements for themselves. They find ways to be better than those around them and usually have a "One Up" story. Pride is said to be the original and most deadly of the seven sins, leading straight to damnation.

The Seven Heavenly Virtues:

Chastity, Abstinence, Liberality, Diligence, Patience, Kindness, Humility.

Chastity- Courage and boldness. Embracing of moral wholesomeness and achieving purity of thought through education and betterment.

Abstinence- Constant mindfulness of others and one's surroundings; practicing self-control, abstention, and moderation.

Liberality- Generosity. Willingness to give. A nobility of thought or actions.

Diligence- A zealous and careful nature in one's actions and work. Decisive work ethic. Budgeting one's time; monitoring one's own activities to guard against laziness.

Patience- Forbearance and endurance through moderation. Resolving conflicts peacefully, as opposed to resorting to violence. The ability to forgive; to show mercy to sinners.

Kindness- Charity, compassion, friendship, and sympathy without prejudice and for its own sake.

Humility- Modest behavior, selflessness, and the giving of respect. Giving credit where credit is due; not unfairly glorifying one's own self. Modest behavior, selflessness, and the giving of respect. Giving credit where credit is due; not unfairly glorifying one's own self.

9

How Spagyric Medicines Work

The spagyric preparations may, in some instances, lead to a healing process stimulated by the body's metabolic response. People may confuse this natural healing process, such as fatigue, stiff and aching joints, or sinus drainage with illness. These symptoms usually indicate that toxins are being eliminated from congested tissue. You're likely to experience these symptoms because the unique synergy of these products works to streamline your rebuilding and elimination, *i.e.*, flush toxins out of the body.

Minerals, trace elements and vitamins are the enablers of metabolism. Carbohydrates, proteins and fats needs them for their synthesis and degradation. The immune system needs them for proper functioning.

As per Biochemistry the human body contains some vital mineral salts, *viz.* calcium, phosphorus, magnesium, iron, sodium, potassium, fluorine, sulphur, chlorine and silicon a deficiency of which disturbs the functions or metabolism.

Trace elements are the activators and co-factors of enzymes and other regulatory molecules, they include selenium, copper, cobalt, iodine, iron, zinc, manganese, vanadium, chromium, boron, chlorine, silicon, fluoride, molybdenum, arsenic, germanium, lithium, nickel, etc.

Trace elements and vitamins work in concert, they are inter-dependent. Effects of trace element deficiencies on living organisms are now accepted by scientists world wide, now a days, faulty agriculture with chemical fertilizers and pesticides, food processing losses and environmental pollution are the basic contributory factors leading to mineral salt deficiencies in living organisms.

The active ingredients in Spagyric Medicines are the mineral salts which function by stimulating neuro immuno endocrine system.

Acccording to Patricia Kaminski and Richard Katz, spagyric essences are among the safest, most self-regulating remedies available. If we take essences that are totally inappropriate and have little relationship to our real issues, then we will experience little effect.

Spagyric essences work by resonance; thus the wrong essences will not stimulate a "soul chord" within us. If we take too many essences, or essences which address only minor issues, they may be ineffective; substantive changes will not be achieved, or will take much longer to occur. Sometimes inappropriate or chaotic essence selections will stimulate confusion or a sense of uneasiness. Perhaps too many issues are "stirred up," or change happens faster than can be tolerated. On occasion, rapid psychological transformation or our resistance to it can produce unpleasant physical sensations such as fatigue, skin rashes, or headaches. Such reactions are generally short-lived, and may be an indication to re-formulate the essence combination, or to work with counseling and other practices to remove any psychological impediments to the therapeutic process.

Because Spagyric essences are something we take into our bodies, it is easy to confuse the essences with drugs which are used to treat physical and emotional illness. Flower essences are not drugs. First of all, because of their vibrational nature, flower essences have no direct impact upon the body's biochemistry, as do pharmaceutical and psychoactive drugs.

Tranquilizers, anti-depressants, pain-killers, mood-brighteners, and "mind- expanding" drugs affect emotional states, but they do this by changing brain chemistry, thus altering the biological vehicle through which the human soul expresses itself.

Such biochemical manipulation may be important in cases of severe illness, such as extreme suicidal tendencies. Yet, apart from the danger of side effects, we must ask profound questions about the use of mood-altering drugs to control or eliminate such typical human emotions as depression, fear, anxiety, and shyness. What is the effect on the soul of chemically-induced personality makeovers? Is something lost when the soul no longer needs to grapple with the pain of childhood abuse, or anger at the injustices of the world?

Can the soul learn life's lessons if it no longer has the freedom to experience pain and transformation? Would society have fared better if its great poets had treated their introversion with mood enhancers, or if its social critics had cured their alienation with anti-depressants?

Spagyric essences, by contrast, leave the soul in freedom. They encourage rather than compel change, working by vibrational resonance rather than bio-chemical intervention. Their effect is evocative, much like the impact of a conversation with a wise and caring friend.

The essences stimulate an inner dialogue with hidden aspects of the Self, awakening profound psychological archetypes, and giving us access to their message. As a result of such "speaking" to our soul, deep emotional and mental changes take place, which may then produce physiological alterations as well. But these changes are not imposed from without; they occur from within ourselves, through our own experience and effort.

Spagyric essences are catalysts which stimulate and energize the inner transformative process, while leaving us free to develop our own innate capacities. They are used best within a context of inner development, through self-observation, dialogue, and counseling.

For this reason, they are not used to treat particular diseases. Rather, flower essences help us to learn the lessons of any ailment, to meet the challenges presented to our souls by emotional and physical pain and suffering, and thus to transform our lives. Such a health-enhancing metamorphosis may naturally eliminate many painful physical symptoms, but the ultimate goal remains the evolution of the soul. Unlike pain-killing or symptom suppressing drugs, which can create long-term dependence when used to control chronic conditions, flower essences stimulate lasting changes in consciousness, which continue to be a part of our lives after we stop taking the essences.

Spagyric essences have much in common with herbal remedies. They share a heritage of using pure ingredients directly from Nature, and a philosophy of working with, rather than suppressing, the healing process.

Spagyric essences are a very specialized form of herbal preparation, which should be distinguished from conventional herbal remedies. Herbal products are made from many parts of the plant, including the root, stem, leaves, fruit, seed, as well as the blossom; they are made by a variety of methods, including infusion, decoction, and tincture.

Spagyric essences differ in their preparation method in that they are generally made by cohobation, and only with the fresh plants within a very specific environmental matrix. In Spagyric essence preparation, the four elements are involved, the earth to nurture the plant; the air from which it feeds; the sun or fire to enable it to impart its power; and water to be enriched with its beneficent magnetic healing. We would also add that there is the fifth alchemical element, the quintessential element, which is the sensitive consciousness of the Spagyric essence preparer. Thus, Spagyric essences are more than simple herbal extracts; they are alchemical quintessences which carry the living archetypes of the whole plant.

Herbal remedies are generally selected on the basis of physical symptoms, and are used for their naturally occurring physical constituents. Spagyric essences, by contrast, are vibrational in nature, and are selected for their impact on soul qualities. Still, within the herbal and shamanic traditions of many cultures there is the knowledge that plants have deeper meanings, and are associated with spiritual forces and processes. This legacy of a more subtle herbalism can be viewed as one of the sources for understanding flower essence qualities.

Often the Spagyric essence's impact on the soul is like a "higher octave" of the physical effects of the plant, although this must be considered in the context of a complete study of the plant. Many modern herbalists use Spagyric essences along with traditional herbal medicaments. However, they report that the essences address issues of the psyche far more directly and precisely than do conventional herbal remedies.

Current scientific research provides explanations for how the remedies act on the body and why they are so effective. The existence of "Water Geometry" as well as water's stability, even after it has been converted into steam, was proven in both Pennsylvania and Berkeley Universities, USA in 1995 and 1996. Following distillation, purification and other productions steps, the plants, minerals and metals are transformed into a spagyric tincture, During the course of the production processes the "life energy" contained within the plant, mineral or metal is released from its attachment to material. This energy, is comprised of three different active energies: Salt, Sulfur, and Mercury. The director of the French Institute for Medicine in Paris, member of the New York Academy of Science and advisor for UNESCO, Louis C Kervran was able to scientifically prove that, specific enzymes cause the transmutation of certain elements such as potassium, hydrogen, magnesium and oxygen into calcium. In the same manner, sodium and hydrogen are transmuted into magnesium, and sodium and oxygen can change into potassium. This phenomenon, which to a certain extent is a natural "alchemical" process, is known as "Biological Transmutation" or the "Kervran Effect".

Research published in the British Homeopathic Journal by Professor R.R. Sharma demonstrated that the energetic information contained in homeopathic medicines is able to cross the blood-brain barrier in a matter of approximately 8 seconds and thus deliver therapeutic effects in a deep manner.

Dr. Peter Schleicher, immunologist from Munich opined, that spagyric medicines are "effective in influencing and activating" PNEI regulation mechanisms. Scientific experiments at the Atomic Institute in Vienna showed that different plants contain different radiation patterns. Every plant possesses a quite individual field of radiation: a particular 'energy fingerprint'. In a fraction of a second this radiation power senses the 'information' embedded in our body's immune system, which is directly linked to the hormone system and connected with emotion.

Spagyric Medicine trigger at this quantum level, and deliver the correct information to activate self-regulation of bodily systems and mechanisms and enhancing its footprint through deep penetration and regulation of cellular functioning which influence at the deepest informational state, respectively the DNAs and RNAs, the higher states of emotional and physical health, thus, influence limbic activity, then hypothalamus and pituitary gland, and finally the sexual organs and adrenal glands, and provides the basis of self-sustainable health.

According to Dr. Peter Schleicher, all levels of this PNI hierarchy can be given regulatory impulses through the help of high quality spagyric medicines.

Even the so-called spontaneous healing of life-threatening diseases such as cancer almost always corresponds with spiritual and mental processes in which there are major changes in the patient's "inner attitude".

From the hermetic point of view; man is, if the Sulfur principle as an immortal part and bearer of the individual "program" (soul) is in unimpeded connection with the mortal principles Salt (body = construction, structure, function, dynamics) and Mercury (spirit = Feeling, feeling, thinking, acting). Man is sick when body and spirit are not connected with the core of the individual soul (Sulfur) and lead a life of their own, which can be seen in signs of illness. This changes Salt (material body) and Mercury (mind).

The Spagyric healing process is analogous to the Spagyric healing process: Spagyry is a reconciliation between the soul's core (Sulfur), the anatomical and physiological structure (Salt), and one's own soul Corresponding feeling and thinking (Mercury).

10

Alchemy and Spagyrics

"Spagyric is the art of looking into the light of nature"

– ***Paracelsus***

Spagyric is an ancient, holistic art of healing. The greek word spagyric is composed of two words, the first one means "breaking„ while the second one means "raising„. Incoporating the 5 elements (earth, water, fire, air and space) with Spagyric plant medicine, body and breathing exercises, healing touch, sounds, defumigation and sacred space.

Spagyric medicine contains aspects of phytotherapy (herbal medicine), homeopathy, aromatherapy and oligotherapy (minerals).

What is the difference between Alchemy and Spagyrics?

Alchemical elixirs are for regeneration, and Spagyric essences or tinctures are for therapeutics.

According to spagyrics and alchemy all substances are mixtures of three basic principle, Sulfur, Mercury and Salt.

Sulphur, the soul of things, in particular of plants, is different for every type of plant. Mercury, the spirit, is the same throughout the plant kingdom, to be specific, it is ethyl alcohol.

Salt, like Sulfur, is characteristic of each type of plant. It is specifically the matrix of the body of the plant.

The first phase of spagyrics consists of separating these principles in their various aspects, while striving to retain their philosophical aspects, *i.e.*, the life forces which they bear.

In the mineral kingdom the life forces are fixed, and only evolve or dissipate very slowly, except human intervention. In the plant kingdom, on the other hand, great variations in the life forces exist. Seeds and fruits, for example, retain their energy for a long time, but while a fresh plant retains almost all of its vital principles, this is not so with a dried plant. In fact, as soon as a plant is detached from it's environment it begins losing its vital principles, hence, in decreasing order of energetic strength, we have the seed or fruit, then the fresh plant, and finally the dried plant (plant dying may, however, produce certain beneficial energetic transformations).

The Separation of the three Principles

First Method: This method is used for fresh or dried plants, or for seeds rich in essential oils, such as, lavender, juniper, rosemary, caraway or cumin.

First Phase: The Extraction of Volatile Sulfur

If the plant used is in the form of a seed, the distillation vase should be a flask, if an entire plant is used, however, a reactor is preferable, as it's large aperture allow the plant to be charged and discharged more easily. The flask itself should be round, in fact, a flask with a flat bottom should not be used with apparatus where work under vacuum might be carried out. The advantage of the vacuum is that the life of the plants and it's principles are easier to handle since the boiling point is lower. Boiling water produces steam which carries alongwith it the essential oil of the plant, it's sulphur. The steam passes through the separator and condense in the cooler.

The lid of the reactor fits on the vat with the help of a flat joint. However, there is one risk here, supposing one is not working under vacuum, then an excessive pressure of steam may occur which, in view of the surface of the lid, is extremely dangerous. For excess pressure of 10cm of water and a lid of 10cm internal diameter, for example, the force pushing the lid will be just over 800g. Consequently, there is a risk of steam escaping through the joint, and the risk of burns. Clearly, the joint itself should be carefully tightened.

The separator has two advantages: first, it makes the collection of the essential oil easier, secondly, the tube which sends the condensation water back to the reactor completely eliminates the risk of running out of water, with its potentially disastrous consequences in this type of distillation.

Caution

If one is working under vacuum, or even if one has not created a vacuum, the tap should never be opened as long as one is uncertain of the balance of internal-external pressures, otherwise the oil could find itself back in the reactor again.

The Manometer

Whether working under vacuum or not, it is advisable to use a vacuum manometer and an anti-return valve. The manometer indicates whether there is a pressure imbalance or not, and hence one could open the tap with ease. The anti-return valve partly prevents an eventual loss of the 'spirits'. In practice one may install a glass on the lateral branch between the anti-return valve and the vacuum grip/outlet on top of the cooler. A small piece of silicon tubing squashed with a pair of pliers is attached for a handle. The slow loosening of the pliers allow the pressure to be equalizes without sudden jumps. The manometer should preferably be the mechanical type, since a mercury manometer requires a fixture which prevents the stem from returning to the installation. Besides, the latter can not accept brutal pressure variations.

The cooler preferably with a straight reflux, or of allihn type, at minimum 50 cm active.

The anti-return valve: a quality valve here will guarantee a vacuum and prevent any risk of explosion, in case of explosion it allows the steam to escape outwards.

The water vacuum horn: stainless steal horns are preferable to all others since they do not very easily. In this process the procedure begins with the extraction of volatile Sulfur, which facilitates it's extraction. However, there is always a significant loss of spirit during this first phase. Once all the oil has been extracted, one should proceed for the next step, *i.e.*, separation of spirit or Mercury.

Second Phase: The Extraction of Mercury

Fermentation

The alcohol produced by fermentation is not found in all the plant kingdom, and becomes determined only in the ensuing operations. In the present case, the steam of the boiling water has destroyed any eventual yeasts in the plant. Besides, it's quite possible that the plant does not posses enough fermentable elements to generate the level of alcohol necessary to extract the mercury. For this reason, the bacterial flora should be reconstituted by adding some brewer's yeast and white sugar or grape sugar. About 1,200 kg of sugar is needed to obtain a liter of alcohol. The amount of alcohol required is 10 and 15 per cent.

Once this is done, the soup thus obtained should be placed in a preferably open recipient of fairly large capacity in order to prevent the fermentation from spilling over.

Place the recipient in a room of about 20° C. At the beginning of the fermentation, put a board or lid upon the recipient to avoid the risk of any rotting. This risk however disappears after 2-3 days. The brew should be stirred every day with a spatula. When during stirring no more gas bubbles rise up to the surface, then the fermentation is complete. The liquid is now separated from the solid for distillation.

In the beginning it is advisable to remove any carbolic gas to increase the reproduction of yeasts, as well as to leave the gas floating on the liquid after two or three days. This will check the multiplication of the yeasts which by this time would spoil the production of alcohol.

Distillation

The globe of kjedahl stops the microbubbles arising due to ebullition. On top, an expansion globe 'cleans up' the vapours, and above all gives the alert distillator much information by the appearance of the liquid veins flowing on the glass. However, this does not make a thermometer dispensable for the work to follow. During fermentation, and especially where stalks are present (*e.g.* with thyme), methylic alcohol is formed. It's name 'wood spirit' explains it's origin. This alcohol is a violent poison which must be removed. It's boiling point is 66.5°C, and it does not create any azeotrope, unlike ethylic alcohol. This means that if to start off the distillation very slow, and all liquid passing when the thermometer reads below 66-67°C is removed, then the methylic alcohol is almost totally eliminated.

Several distillations are required to bring the alcohol-mercury to the desired degree, and if these are properly carried out, *i.e.* very slowly, the residue in methylic alcohol will be negligible. The vacuum faucet/tap/plug is designed to avoid excessively high pressure, and it is conveniently plugged up by a stopper made of loose cotton wool. All distillations should cease as soon as the thermometer registers 85°C. Distillation under vacuum requires a different type of apparatus to be workable in practice.

We have now obtained the volatile Sulfur and the Mercury. There now remains the distilled fermented liquid, as well as the solid residue separated before the distillation.

Third Phase: The Extraction of Fixed Sulfur or Salt of Sulfur

A new distillation is carried out with the newly distilled liquid, and this time the temperature should reach 100°C. The water and phlegms thus obtained should be set aside for the work on the salts, and it is best to distill the water a second time for this work.

As soon as the liquid looks like honey, the first distillation should be stopped, otherwise it becomes impossible to take the 'honey' out of the flask. The drying process should be completed gradually in a crucible in open air. If the honey is completely dry, and if the plant is thought to contain volatile salts, then it should be calcined in a closed luted crucible. During this calcinations a fixture is required to prevent the lid of the crucible from rising, and a few hours at 400°C should be enough. The heating should be done at the base of the crucible to allow the volatile salts to lay down on the inside of the lid. Good experience is required for this operation to succeed. The residual honey should then be calcined, as described. However, if the honey is not perfectly dry, or if it is thought that there are no volatile salts, or the residue from the proceeding operation is taken, the following procedure then be adopted. The carbon should be eliminated by causing combustion through oxygen from air(which previously was not possible in the closed crucible), *i.e.*, one should operate with an open crucible. As soon as the honey is in a solid state, it is reduced to powder as finely as possible. For the calcination of this powder, 400°C suffice, as long as the stirring instrument is made of pyrex glass.

Next, when the powder is greyish white, it is washed in small extractor in the soxhlet. Once extracted, in this washing of the salt and in all others to follow, the charge water of the soxhlet is the water obtained through distillation of the soup after extraction of the mercury. The solution is then slowly evaporated, and the salt crystals are obtained.

At this point of operation, we have the following:

A rectified Mercury

A volatile Sulfur (essential oil)

A volatile Salt of Sulfur (the salt from the top of crucible)

A fixed and soluble Salt of Sulfur (resulting from the coagulation of the extraction of the soxhlet)

Fourth Phase: the Extraction of the Fixed Salt of the Plant

At this point the solid part separated from the soup should be calcined in an open crucible. Certain schools advise placing a large funnel above the crucible to collect and condense the first smoke issuing from the calcinations. The deposits thus obtained can only be recouped by a dissolution in alcohol. Once the alcohol has been evaporated and coagulation has taken place, one obtains a substance which represents the remains of the fixed sulphuric salt in the solid part of the plant. If one is able to purify this matter, either by solve-coagula with the alcohol, or by distillation, then one can mix it with the fixed salt of sulphur. This is a delicate procedure, however, requiring some experience.

The coal like residue is powdered as fine as possible in the air until it is grayish- white. Next, it is extracted in the soxhlet. The solid part remaining in the cartridge after an eventual final calcination is the fixed insoluable salt. The extraction water is slowly evaporated, and the fixed soluble salt will be obtained. If this salt is not absolutely white, if it is not hydroscopic, and if the extraction water is coloured, then one has to begin the cycle all over again.

All the principles of the plant are now separated as below:

The volatile Sulfur

The salt of the volatile Sulfur

The salt of the fixed soluble Sulfur

The salt of the fixed insoluble Sulfur

Mercury

Fixed soluble salt

Fixed insoluble salt

Generally speaking, the insoluble salts are now utilized and are considered *caput mortem*.

There now follows the cohobation or reunion of the principles.

The Seperation of the Principles

Second Method

First Phase: The Preparation of the Alcohol

This alcohol should only be derived from red wine, since here none of the advantages of alcohol being produced during fermentation are present.

The wine should be distilled, as before, everything passing over before the steam has reached 76-77°C is discarded, and the distillation is stopped at 85°C. The distillates are collected and distilled once more. This process is repeated until the alcohol has alcohol level exceeding 90 per cent. From this moment onwards, although the increase of alcoholic degrees after each distillation is slight, the distillations should nevertheless be continued until some drops of greenish yellow oil appear on the surface of the fluid. This oil, called 'death principles' should be discarded.

There are now three possible ways of proceeding:

1. The alcohol of 92-93° may be used with certain precautions.
2. The quality of the alcohol may be improved by vacuum distillation.
3. The alcohol may be treated with potassium carbonate.

Vacuum Distillation

Since this is a delicate process, its best to use only for rectification, *i.e.*, after at least the third or fourth distillation. The great difficulty that vacuum distillation presents is that the liquid to be distilled tends to jump around widely, thus passing directly into the receptor flask. On the other hand, we need not be concerned with the distillation stones or the capillary tube for constant air injection, both of which stabilise the distillation process. This is because both these fixtures require constant maintenance of the vacuum, which is only obtainable by an extremely expensive vacuum pump.

Because of the 'thrusts' of the liquid take place suddenly, the reversed flask on top of the distillation flask can absorb a great part of the flow of liquid bubbles. The part that is that is not stopped by this fixture enters the lateral tubing which, together with the globe of khedahl, constitutes a second wall for stopping the flux of bubbles. The residue should be stopped by expansion globe on top of the sphere of khedahl. If the furnace is carefully monitored, it is possible to successfully distill with this apparatus.

Note: the temperature indicated on the thermometer is lower than that in the current distillation. Also, the manometer and the anti-return valve are indispensable here. The limit of the alcoholic degree through vacuum distillation is 99.5°, but a net result of 98° or above is also fine.

Distillation of Calcined Tarter

Alchemically speaking, this process has the reputation of 'mineralising' alcohol. Once the alcohol has exceeded 92-93°, this process consists of setting It to macerate with calcined potassium carbonate. The latter is very hydrophyllic and absorbs the water content of the alcohol. The maceration is then carefully distilled, it yields an alcohol of between 98-99.9°.

It is true enough that often, before the last distillation, one may notice a yellowish discoloration of the alcohol, leading one to conclude that it has extracted a 'mineral tincture' from the carbonate. However, if one bears in mind that, on the other hand, potassium carbonate is very often the major element of plant salt, then one has good reason to believe that the use of alcohol that has been distilled with tartar in spagyric operations only represents a minor inconvenience.

Second Phase: The Separation of the Principles

The most vital tool here is a soxhlet extractor or kumagawa extractor. The extraction liquid is poured into the lower flask, here, an alcohol of a quality relative to the desired result is also poured in. A cartridge filled with the plant matter to be extracted is placed in the extraction chamber.

The alcohol end sup in the lower flask, and the vapours pass into the soxhlet through the lateral tube (in kumagawa they pass along the sides of the cartridge). In both cases, the vapours arrive in the cooler, condense, and fall into the cartridge.

From this point and onwards, the cartridge needs to be constantly fed with distilled alcohol. As soon as the level of this alcohol reaches the upper level on top of the syphon, the latter *primes itself* (s'amorace), and the alcohol flows down into the lower flask. Every time the syphon *primes itself* (s'amorace) the colour of the alcohol in the syphon is trans parent again, the extraction is complete.

Two things should be noted for operation to be successfully completed. First, if a weak alcohol of 80-90° is used, and if the furnace is handled cautiously, then the alcohol alone will pass over. In fact, the extraction will then be the same as that using a higher degree alcohol, although water will be present in the tincture nevertheless.

Secondly, the kumagawa extractor has the advantage of having an internal syphon, making extractions possible which are quite not performable with the soxhlet. For example, whereas gummy and crystalline substances such as those yielded by *Harpagophytum* and wine tartar will block the syphon of the soxhlet, this will not occur with the kumagawa in which the syphon is maintained at the same temperature as the vapours. Nevertheless, this inconvenience may be reduced and even eliminated by enclosing it with the thermal insulation(two or three layers of paper) in such a way that the heat emanating from the top of the flask maintains the syphon at an adequate temperature. The solid dregs remaining in the cartridge after extraction are treated by calcinations and solve-coagula, as in the first method in the section dealing with the fixed salt of plants.

At the end of the second phase, we obtain a tincture comprising;

The Sulfur and the Mercury

A fixed soluble Salt

A fixed insoluble Salt

In this method, although the tincture contains some volatile Sulfur and some Mercury, the link between the two principles is so strong that separating them and retrieving the Sulphur through distillation of the tincture is practically impossible.

The Various Spagyric Preparations

These preparations are obtained starting from the separated principles. The most appropriate process of preparation should be choosen depending on the desired product and the intended use.

Tinctures

These are extracts containing the Sulfur and the Mercury without the Salt. The second method is better suited for these preparations. The liquid obtained from the soxhlet or kumagawa extractor is a perfectly acceptable tincture.

A simpler way of extracting a tincture is to put the plant in digestion with a suitable alcohol in an airtight jar. In this case, however, the tincture only reaches full value and potency after several months of digestion.

In tinctures, the curative properties of the plant are exalted. However, in contrast to the elixirs or the essences, the eventually toxic aspects of the plant are not mitigated.

Essences

An essence, or Mercury, or Spirit is obtained by using the first method of distilling and rectifying the fermented liquid. If the second method is used, it is obtained by distillation of the tincture. In both methods, the distillation thus obtained is never toxic as long as the methylic alcohol is eliminated. The therapeutic effects of the essences are more subtle and spiritual than those of tinctures.

While tinctures are suitable for treating physical ailments, essences are rather effective on the emotional and mental levels.

The alcohol or essence obtained through distillation of the tincture is now determined, since it is carrier for the air and water energies of the plant. The essence thus obtained will keep well, but it is still possible to modify it's action through the following methods.

The spiritual potency of a tincture is increased by dissolving it in some of the Sulphur of the plant, either in the form of essential oil, or in the form of Sulphur Salt. In the latter, the tincture should contain about 30 per cent water to allow the Sulphur Salt to be dissolved. The simplest way of doing this is to perform the extraction with alcohol brought to 70°, or to add 30 per cent distilled water to the essence.

Note: The use of alcohol of 70° may cause the Salt to be brought into the tincture if the extraction is not properly conducted. The essence with 30 per cent water may be used to treat physical ailments by dissolving the fixed soluble salt of the plant in it.

Essential Oils

The extraction of the essential oil, or the Sulphur is done according to the first method as discussed in the first phase.

Caution: several essential oils are toxic to various degrees, even in small doses, therefore, one should not utilize these pure essential oils without consulting good literatures on the subject (Essential Oils by Gunther, and Medicinal and Toxic Plants by Fournier, etc.).

Elixirs

These are tinctures that have been purified by the action of the Salt. Salt, while being the main vehicle for the toxic elements, is also the purifying element. A tincture may be transformed into an elixir by the circulation of the tincture on the Salt, using either the slow method with the meeting vases or the pelican, or the rapid method which consists of placing the tincture and the Salt in a flask topped by a cooler, after which an ongoing auto-distillation is carried out. After several hours, the Salt absorbs the impurities, and once saturated with it the operation should be stopped, and the tincture of the Salt separated. The latter should then be calcined to remove any impurities in it. If it does not become white, again a solve-coagula should be carried out on it, and the circulation also. The Salt used in this procedure is the fixed soluble Salt.

After the circulation, the separation can be carried out either by filtering or by distillation. Filtering is preferable since the distillation is injurious to the Sulphur of the tincture. This process should be continued as long as the Salt becomes coloured. Theoretically, the separation of the principles is not total, and the circulation of the tincture-Salt, in it's initial stages, will continue this separation. Since the discolouration of the tincture only begins after the complete separation, it is possible that during the two or three initial circulations the tincture becomes coloured rather than discoloured. The symbolism involve here is noteworthy: it is fire and water which purify the Salt. Twenty to thirty circulations, or even more may be necessary.

The Circulation of the Stones

The processes are identical for both preparations. It is simply the weight ratio between the essence and the Salt which determines the emphasis, which is either circulatus-liquid stone or solid stone.

The circulates has great extracting power, but only weak spagyric healing potentials. To obtain these two preparations, the first method of separation is preferable by far.

First, all the volatile and fixed Sulphurs should be collected with the exception of the fixed insoluble Sulphur. Only the fixed Salt is utilized. It is important here to remember that the vital energies can only be accumulated in the liquid or soluble bodies, and are fixed by the solid state. It is by joining the totality of the Sulphurs that the philospical Sulphur is reestablished. That is to say, the Salt of Sulphur is dissolved in the volatile Sulphur. With this Sulphur the fixed Salt is soaked up. As soon as the Salt is dry, it is soaked up more and more until it will absorb no more. There should never be any flowing liquid during these soakings. From this moment onwards we have the choice of either circulates or solid stone.

The Circulates or Liquid Stone

The Salt is saturated with a quantity of essence (the rectified essence of the plant) between 10 to 15 times that of the Salt. These circulations should be followed by distillations in order to cause the separation, and then a new uniting and another circulation. This circulation is often called cohobation. The alcohol should become acid after six or seven circulations. The test of a finished circulates is that it should immediately decompose fresh vegetable material, after that it may be recouped through distillation.

The Solid Stone

To obtain the solid stone, the Sulfur saturated Salt should be soaked with Mercury with the latter becoming runny. Only the surface of the Salt should become moist. This soaked Salt is put in an incubator at 40°C. Soaking should take place about once a week until it will absorb absolutely no more, and set in the incubator. The stone is a real success if the Salt meets these three criteria:

1. A consistency like wax
2. Is insoluable in water
3. Will fuse easily and without any smoke

There are numerous plants which will allow these results without too much difficulty: caraway, celandine, lavender and thyme, for instance. It may also be obtained by the combination of tincture of wheat and cream of tartar. Great care should be taken to look out for possible bacterial contamination, as well as contamination due to parasite Sulphur during the process of stone or circulatus.

The Acetone of the Ancients

According to Becker, the red oil extracted from acetone of the ancients is an excellent remedy of a universal character. The process of extracting it is here greatly modified. According to the ancients, the substance most full of 'vital spirit' is sea salt and the acid derived from it. Sea salt is the most important mineral in human blood, but it is not actually used in our operation.

One should obtain limestone recently obtained from the sea, the simplest and surest being oyster shell.

Preparation of the Shells

These should be cleaned in a dry condition by rubbing and scouring them in order to remove any animal or vegetable residue fro the shell. Washing them in water may weaken the vital principles with which oyster shell has impregnated itself through the action of the sea salt. The shells are then ground. It is not necessary to grind them very finely, and granules of 1 to 2 mm size are perfectly acceptable. The shells and wine vinegar are the only ingredients required.

Preparation of the Vinegar

Red wine vinegar in plastic bottles only should be bought, and emptied out to one-fifth or one quarter of their volume. They are then placed in a deep freezer of an optimum temperature of -25°C(at -18°C the process of separation will be slower to take off). If the bottles are made of glass or if they are partially empty, they will explode under the effect of the expansion of the vinegar while freezing.

The active element of vinegar is acetic acid. If one takes pure water and adds acetic acid, the freezing point of the mixture will be lower, and a maximum of 60 per cent acid at about-25°C. If the percentage of acid increases, the freezing point will climb up to 0°C, and for pure acid it is at 17°C.

After twenty four hours of remaining in the freezer, the vinegar is almost completely frozen solid. The bottle is then placed upside -down on top of a phial of the Erlenmeyer type. A red liquid will start flowing out, and one stops as soon as the ice block becomes white or pale pink, the latter is discarded since there is no acid left in it.

All the red liquids are collected, and one starts again. Next, the red liquids of the second freezing are distilled, stopping as soon as the liquid takes on colour. In this way a vinegar of density between 1,040 and 1,060 is obtained, one which is suitable for the rest of our operations.

One must keep in mind that vinegar is less rich in acetic acid than wine is in alcohol. Common vinegar generally consists 65 acid by volume. Taking a 1 per cent loss in account, which is very little, then 20 liters of vinegar are required for 1 liter of pure acid.

Now that our two base substances are ready, a soxhlet is filled with the oyster shells in the cartridge, and the lower flask is filled with the distilled vinegar. The top of the cooler should not be stopped up, as some amount of gas is liable to escape during the extraction. The shells should gradually dissolve in the vinegar. If crystals should appear in the flask, the extraction should be stopped, and the apparatus is allowed to cool off. The crystals will begin to form. These should be separated from the liquid by decantation. It is not imperative to use the soxhlet for dissolving the shells, but in this case it becomes necessary to decant and filter the solution very carefully.

The vinegar coming from the decantation is complemented with fresh vinegar, and the extraction is continued. In the end, one part of vinegar should be distilled, one third of it's volume, for instance.

With cooling, crystals will form, and these are separated. A third of the remaining vinegar is distilled again, yielding new crystals, and so on.

In modern terminology, the crystals are calcium acetate. As soon as a few crystal have been obtained, they are put a side in an airtight jar because the added infusion (*surfusion*) or the refusal (*refus*) of crystallization commonly occurs with acetates. As soon as the vinegar from the extraction is cooled, and if it no longer crystallizes, then a tiny piece of crystal, obtained previously, should be thrown into the liquid. If acetate forms, crystallization occurs in just a few seconds.

The calcium acetate thus prepared is placed in a flask preferably made of sandstone, since the dry distillation of calcium acetate badly damages flasks made of glass.

The condensation of the vapours from the dry distillation will yield acetone with a temperature of 56.3°C. Everything passing over before 54°C and after 60°C should be discarded. A second distillation of the acetone is then required.

The acetone is placed in a decanting phial or in some such piece of equipment. Complete water-tightness is required here, since, this alone will prevent the acetone from evaporating. The free surface of the liquid should also be rather large. At the end of a time period between one and six months, a sheath of red liquid should completely cover the acetone, which is called the red oil. The acetone is then withdrawn, and the red oil is then left in the ampule. Just enough absolute alcohol is then poured into the ampule which is then spread over the entire surface of the glass to dissolve the oil sticking to it.

This alcohol is a powerful remedy. The dose depends on the concentration of alcohol- oil, but in general, a few drops in half a glass of water will be plenty. Becker says that its action is universal enough and close to that attributed to Paracelsus and other's tincture of pearls. Cleopatra is said to have drunk vinegar in which pearls have been dissolved.

The Significance of Metals

The concept of metal, in Alchemy and Spagyria, is directly linked to of 'mineral ontogeny mechanisms, that the Ancients defined the parameters through more or less clarifying symbolic matrices.

The genesis of the metals within the bowels of the earth was the 'original act that is found in their own organic projection in the structure of 'man; The humoral theory it is an example. The man, as a whole undivided, is a secondary analogatum of supreme analogate cosmic: there is interaction because all the objective identified are linked by similar processes subsistence (basic assumption of Paracelsus).

It is therefore important to the metal itself, considered as a pure element interacting in pharmacodynamic level, but complexifications that contains it, or complessificazioni resulting therefrom.

It is in the mutual interaction between the different constituents of the activated complex and dynamic that we find the 'Metal Action on re-organic functional balance, and not in the symbolic specificities linked to more or less obscure planetary aspects. If there is a metal-planet interaction, according to the dictates of the traditional Spagyria, this is only archetypal than the actual dynamics of Spagyrico drug. Still, the 'analogy planetary assumes when integrated value in the microcosm-macrocosm dictated that all 'vintage replaced the 'current and accurate scientific experimental conceptualization.

In this table we can observe a general relationship between metal-physiological and pathological structure, as well as modern science has experimental Spagyric able to define (consider the non-exclusivity of systematization):

Oro	Spleen
(Gold)	SNC
	Circulatory system
	Visual apparatus
	Heart diseases and related diseases
	Alzheimers diseases
	Arthritis, degenerative diseases
	Hypogammaglobulinemia
Argento	Esophagus, stomach, channel intestinal
(Silver)	Thyroid
	breast Giandole
	Uterus and ovaries (function women in general)
	Lymphatic system
	joint lubrication
	Amenorrhea and false
	menopause
	tinnitus
	Epilepsy
	Edemas in the upper limbs. and/or inf.
	Insomnia of nervous origin
	heart palpitations
	Dizziness
Stagno	Liver
(Tin)	Arteries and blood flow
	Adrenal glands
	assimilation and enrichment of blood
	Immune system

	carbohydrate metabolism
	tissue generation
	genito-urinary organs
	respiratory system
	All specific diseases connected thereto
Ferro	blood biochemical processes
(Iron)	liver biochemical processes
	motor nerves
	genitals
	rectum
	combustion processes
	fibrous tissue
	Dysentery and obstructions
	liver, spleen and mesentery
	Fluxions blood
	Gonorrhea
	Fluxions belly of hemorrhoids and menstruation
	Anemia
	Serum iron, breakthrough bleeding, spermatorrhea
Mercurio	Organs of 'hearing, taste and vocal organs
(Mercury)	peripheral nervous system the liquid circulation
	cerebrospinal respiratory system
	Diseases of the peripheral nerves
	Plexus disorders
	bronchial asthenia
	Headache and nerve disorders
	Inflammation of apparatus respiratory
Piombo	Heart and circulatory system
(Lead)	myocardial muscle and endocardium
	Bones and calcium balance

	joints
	Spleen
	Mineral adjustment in blood
	cardiovascular diseases
	Osteoporosis, forms arthritic and rheumatic
	Diathesis spleen contractions
	Stiffening and calcification tendon
Rame	Connective tissue
(Copper)	Reproductive physiology muscles
	Kidney and renal papillae
	Thymus and Thyroid diuretics and function processes blood
	Internal organs generators
	Continued fevers and intermittent
	Kidney diseases
	muscle and tendon pain
	Pathologies of 'apparatus reproductive accumulation of cholesterol

TABLES OF METAL STRUCTURES PHYSIOLOGICAL REFERENCE PATHOLOGY

The study of the correlation is significant when integrated to 'inside of a system valid scientific, where the 'investigation is not a' random gamble but a real commitment towards a rebalancing of the structures offended by the disease.

Identified the 'body or the main function affected, there are complex mineral or vegetable specifically active at various levels of the human microcosm a corollary to the influence of the macrocosm. Each one of the base metals has some complementary to it closely related that serve to complete, improve and individualize the individual patient therapy.

The basic therapeutic choice is automatic, but the choice of complexes with complementary ingredients requires consultation of the materia medica spagyrical. It will be choice also the dilution and the mode of administration of the metal that will vary second concentration of the organic and of the need for the specific metal.

The planetary type fits here as structural analogy and not as real influence; therefore, the patient of a certain planet (to use a terminology common) will be much more sensitive to its metal, the more is uncontrolled and in these cases tolerate only infinitesimal doses of this. The subject in good health takes advantage of his metal trace element, will have on him a powerful stimulating effect on viability, but the ill have to always receive very high doses.

In the table below you can see a greater systematization of correlations between metals and internal physiological structures; you can see here the prominence of targeted action:

METAL STRUCTURES PHYSIOLOGICAL REFERENCE PATHOLOGY

Au- Heart, stomach, duodenum, Gonads

Ag- autonomic nervous system

Hg- Central nervous system, Lungs

Cu- Excretory system, reproductive

Fe- Gall bladder, small intestine, Colon

Sn- Liver

Pb- Spleen and immune system

Sb- Pancreas

In addition, each disease has specific features and finds a match Analog-to psychological level of human types:

METAL STRUCTURES PHYSIOLOGICAL REFERENCE PATHOLOGY

Au- Energy, boost growth

Ag- Hypersensitivity, conditionability

Hg- Instability, transience

Cu- Acceptance, openness

Fe- Contrast, hardness

Sn- Balance, accumulation

Pb- Stubbornness, determination

Clearly the pathologies are not dependent on any planetary influence or cosmic imbalance, but only by organic interaction factors that produce in certain cases the onset of disequilibrium factors at the level of five elements set out above. we will have therefore:

METALS PATHOLOGICAL TYPES

Au- Pathologies with underdevelopment, degeneration or atrophy of specific organs

Ag- Pathologies resulting from alteration of nervous tissue

Hg- mental illness

Cu- Pathologies that tend to progress or recur for deficient defenses immunological

Fe- acute inflammatory diseases with lively organic reactivity

Sn - Diseases characterized by 'accumulation and deposit of toxins

Pb- Estremememente serious diseases per se (Neoplasms) for immunological deficit stabilized

Sb- Disorders of hepato-pancreatic level spleen, where necessary a strong cleansing.

Interesting to note is now the relationship that each has with those groups of Metal chemical elements whose pharmacodynamic behavior affects relations between the organs and the endocrine system 3. Without going into detail too much, we affirm a character particularly existing dynamic interrelation between the endocrine system and internal organs.

Below we can see the relationship table:

METALS AND RELATED ELEMENTS

Au- S, Na, Si, Pt, Sb

Ag- Cr, Mn, P, Pd

Hg- It should, I, Se, Ge

Cu- Zn, Br, K, F

Fe- As, Co, Al

Sn- Ca, Li, Mg, Ni

Pb- Ba, Cd, Bi

The organs are in binary equilibrium: each organ corresponds to a structure endocrine presiding over its function. The greater the 'activities of' organ, the lesser is that of endocrine structure, all with a mechanism of feedback.

L 'epiphysis works much when the immune heritage is being formed, then atrophied to the maturation of this; however useful is its stimulation in case of lesions indicating a severe immune impairment. Each pair organ - gland.

It corresponds to a precise function that the specific gland stimulates el 'organ attributed realizes. Therefore, the 'hypothalamus coordinates all functions that support life, while the bark elaborates and realizes. Everything is perceived at the hypothalamic level, relation to stimuli from the soma, as the need for food, to make a example; the cerebral cortex then processes all the mechanisms in order to provide nourishment to 'body.

L 'hypothalamus acts as a sensor to organic needs and transmits to the cortex. All a number of diseases are presented as expressions of alterations of this axis that It should be in balance but in reality is never that.

A non-execution of the hypothalamic instructions from the bark therefore determines unrest, but if the hypothalamic message a lot We ignored we will have a 'structural alteration of the cortex, but no longer directly in correlation with its trophic-regulatory body: thus determining the manifestations clinics as neurosis, psychosis, etc.

The deficient hypothalamic function can lead to a certain decline of brain structures that will be more exposed to noxious stimuli also infections, such as meningitis and similar. If the 'alteration becomes permanent it will be highlighted whenever the body, he is experiencing a particularly difficult time'.

The gradual exclusion of the hypothalamic pulse determines pathologies increasingly deep, up to the degeneration of the nervous system. In this case the therapy will be of sedation of hypothalamic responsiveness, steps at which an efficient nervous system can cater to all its requests and reinforcing stimulus.

The same applies to the thymus, other particularly important gland. Every serious problem of 'respiratory system is often connected with a hypofunction thymus. This gland has features that go far beyond the immunological stimulation, conditioning in general the perfusion is the process of tissue oxygenation. His excessive Operating results in an interesting stimulus on 'cardiovascular system with reactive hypertension and, in the nervous system, depression prone to phobias; her hypofunction determines sclerosis tissue perfusion and tendency to degeneration.

A fundamental and little-known difference exists between carcinomas supported by a deficit epiphyseal (related to issues allergic-iperergiche) and carcinomas supported from a thymic deficits (related to damage of perfusion and tissue oxygenation) and, still, cancers related to a pituitary deficiency (related to issues of nutrition and of tissue protein stores).

In this game of interrelations it is not to forget the possibility of the remedy Spagyrico, who does not want to take the place of traditional medicine, but open the possibility of a fruitful collaboration in research devoted to a broader vision of 'universe Man.

Gem Elixirs

Alchemical elixirs of metals, monoatomic elements, gems and minerals have a long tradition of use for transformation by the initiate few. These elixirs are also understood to be the capstone of the natural healing arts.

First Stage

A particular gem, mineral or rock is selected.

Second Stage

The internal, crystalline structure of the gemstone has been destroyed; the formerly hard stone has been turned into a brittle mass that is easily broken by hand. Such a transformation is usually accompanied by a change in color. This is the first step in manufacturing a truly alchemical preparation: In alchemy, we postulate that every created thing, no matter if it is a rock, a plant, or an animal, is permeated and held together by the creative energies or by the nonphysical conceptual blueprint specific to the material at hand. Steiner called this the "formative forces". In alchemy, it is simply called "spirit". In alchemical literature, we find the Latin instruction: solve et coagula, which stands for "dissolve and coagulate". Its deeper meaning is to dissolve the body, and to coagulate or capture the spirit. At this stage, the gemstone has undergone the first "dissolution".

Third Stage

A look at the flask as we take it out of the incubator, after it has been exposed to at least six weeks of gentle heat. The gemstone had to undergo several treatments to arrive at this stage: The brittle mass of stage two shown in the Obsidian picture sequence was reacted with a plant-derived salt. This reaction is achieved by high temperature cooking, reminiscent of preparing a crème anglaise. The purpose of this step is to further dissolve the material into nanometer-sized clusters, and to prepare the compound for taking up the so-called spiritus mundi, which translates as "spirit of the world". In alchemy, we do not engage in the academic discussion whether the "ether of the ancients" does exist or not, we put it to use. This is the ancient and still secret technology at the core of our manufacturing process. We let the solvent extract the formative forces of the gemstone or mineral. The liquid thus obtained is a carrier of a nonphysical component, aptly called the etheric part or spirit, which interacts directly with the human mind on an etheric level. In alchemical literature, this extraction technique is called circulation or simply fermentation.

Fourth Stage

The liquid obtained from circulation is alcohol and pH adjusted and submitted to cold plasma treatment for further enhancement. The microclusters of the gemstone expand into the now lesser dense solvent, forming a supersaturated solution/suspension in what has now become the so-called mother tincture.

Fifth Stage

The finished product, the gem elixir in homeopathic potency 1X. Ancient alchemical texts suggest dilutions of up to 1:40. In alignment with modern homeopathy, we dilute the mother tincture only at a ratio of 1:9 to obtain the homeopathic potency 1X. This means one part of the mother tincture is diluted and succused (vigorously shaken) with nine parts of distilled water and alcohol. At this low dilution, the finished elixir still contains more microclusters than the solvent can hold in solution, a precipitate is present, hence, shaking the bottle once before taking the elixir is advised.

Elixir of Gold

The following uses for gold are gathered from a number of sources as well as from anecdotal comments. Gold has been used for centuries for jewellery and decoration. In addition to the more familiar rings, brooches, necklaces, and ear rings, gold is used as gold leaf for decoration and protection, screen printing (directly on to bone china, earthenware, porcelain, and glass surfaces or decals). Gold is the key component for "liquid gold", preparations containing up to 12 per cent gold ideal for decorative application using brushes and gold pastes used for screen printing. Gold is also well known as a coinage metal (because of its scarcity, inertness, and decorative features) and is a standard for monetary systems in many countries. Apart from gold coins, gold ingots, and gold bars, gold is available in many forms including pure gold and alloys as gold flakes, foil gauzes (meshes), grain, powders, sheet, sponges, tubes, wires and even single gold crystals.

Recently, gold catalysts as gold supported on carbon or metal oxides are becoming useful in the chemical industry. Many other gold compounds including neutral gold halides ($AuBr3$, etc.), aurates ($K[AuBr4]$, etc.) gold cyanides, gold oxides, phosphine gold complexes, gold hydroxides and gold nitrates are available to industrial users. Chlorauric acid ($HAuCl4$) is used in photography for toning the silver image.

Gold is a really useful metal for electronics because of its inertness and physical properties. Gold is used for electrical contacts, spring contacts, bonding wire, solder alloys, bonding wire, bumping wire, electroplating, and sputtering targets. Gold is also a useful brazing material. Gold is used for coating space satellites, as it is a good IR reflector and is inert.

Since gold is inert and possesses useful properties when alloyed, gold is used extensively for dentistry in gold teeth, dental attachments, inserts, and solders. Similarly, gold is used increasingly for medical implants in eyes and ears, as well as many other medically useful wires, tubes, sheets, and foils. Disodium aurothiomalate is administered (intramuscular) as a treatment for arthritis. The gold isotope 198Au is used for treating cancer and other conditions.

Gold is used in nanotechnology applications as colloids, conjugates, nanoparticle inks, nanoparticle solutions, and nanopowders.

Geological Information

Abundances

In this table values are given in units of ppb (parts per billion; 1 billion = 109), both in terms of weight and in terms of numbers of atoms. Values for abundances are difficult to determine with much certainty, so all values should be treated with some caution, especially so for the less common elements. Local concentrations of any element can vary from those given here by orders of magnitude.

Abundance	*ppb by Weight*	*ppb by Atoms*
Universe	0.6	0.004
Sun	1	0.01
Meteorite (carbonaceous)	170	20
Crustal rocks	3.1	0.3
Sea water	0.05	0.0016
Stream	0.002	0.00001
Human	100	3

Notes

Gold is found as the free element in nature and associated with quartz, pyrite and other minerals. Two thirds of the world's supply comes from South Africa. Much of the USA production is from the states South Dakota and Nevada. Gold is found in sea water (about 5-6 g in a million tonnes of seawater), but no effective economic process has been designed (yet) to extract it from this source.

Historical Information

Discovered by:	Known since ancient times.
Discovered at:	not known
Discovered when:	no data

Origin of name: From the Anglo-Saxon word "gold" (the origin of the symbol Au is the Latin word "aurum" meaning "gold")

Notes

Gold was known and highly valued from earliest times. Egyptian inscriptions dating back to 2600 B.C. describe gold and gold is mentioned several times in the Old Testament.

Gold is one of the elements which has an alchemical symbol, shown below (alchemy is an ancient pursuit concerned with, for instance, the transformation of other metals into gold).

Sometime prior to the autumn of 1803, the Englishman John Dalton was able to explain the results of some of his studies by assuming that matter is composed of atoms and that all samples of any given compound consist of the same combination of these atoms. Dalton also noted that in series of compounds, the ratios of the masses of the second element that combine with a given weight of the first element can be reduced to small whole numbers (the law of multiple proportions). This was further evidence for atoms. Dalton's theory of atoms was published by Thomas Thomson in the 3rd edition of his System of Chemistry in 1807 and in a paper about strontium oxalates published in the Philosophical Transactions. Dalton published these ideas himself in the following year in the New System of Chemical Philosophy.

(History of Chemistry, Sir Edward Thorpe, volume 1, Watts and Co, London, 1914)

Gold has been the basis of many currencies over the centuries and so for economic reasons, among others, the possession of gold was or is restricted in some countries. Notably, private ownership of gold (apart from as jewelry and coins) was banned between 1933 and 1975.

Biological Information

Biological Role

Here are a few notes about the biological role of gold.

Gold has no biological role but does form the basis of some drugs (possibly toxic) used to treat rheumatoid arthritis. Its mode of action appears not to be understood.

Levels in Humans

The following gives the abundances of the elements in humans.

Human abundance [/ppb by weight]: 100

Human abundance [/atoms (C = 1000000)]: 3

Hazards and Risks

Here are a few notes about the hazards and risks associated with gold.

Gold is not absorbed well by the body and its compounds are not normally particularly toxic. Up to 50 per cent of arthritic patients treated with gold-containing drugs may show toxic effects however resulting in damage to the liver and to the kidneys.

Chemical Reactions of the Elements

Reaction of Gold with Air

Gold metal is stable in air under normal conditions. However gold does dissolve in aqueous cyanide solutions in the presence of air.

Reaction of Gold with Water

Gold does not react with water.

Reaction of Gold with the Halogens

Gold metal reacts with chlorine, Cl_2, or bromine, Br_2, to form the trihalides gold(III) chloride, $AuCl_3$, or gold(III) bromide, $AuBr_3$, respectively. On the other hand, gold metal reacts with iodine, I_2, to form the monohalide gold(I) chloride, AuI.

$2Au(s) + 3Cl_2(g) \rightarrow 2AuCl_3(s)$

$2Au(s) + 3Br_2(g) \rightarrow 2AuBr_3(s)$

$2Au(s) + I_2(g) \rightarrow 2AuI(s)$

Solutions of chlorine, Cl_2, and trimethylammonium chloride, $[NHMe_3]Cl$, in acetonitrile, MeCN, dissolve gold.

Reaction of Gold with Acids

Gold metal dissolves in aqua regia, a mixture of hydrochloric acid, HCl, and concentrated nitric acid, HNO_3, in a 3:1 ratio. The name aqua regia was coined by alchemists because of its ability to dissolve gold - the "king of metals".

Reaction of Gold with Bases

Gold does not react with aqueous bases.

Binary Compounds

This section lists some binary compounds with halogens (known as halides), oxygen (known as oxides), hydrogen (known as hydrides), and some other compounds of gold. For each compound, a formal oxidation number for gold is given, but the usefulness of this number is limited for p-block elements in particular. Based upon that oxidation number, an electronic configuration is also given but note that for more exotic compounds you should view this as a guide only. The term hydride is used in a generic sense to indicate compounds of the type M_xH_y and not necessarily to indicate that any compounds listed behave chemically as hydrides.

In compounds of gold (where known), the most common oxidation numbers of gold are: 3.

Hydrides

The term hydride is used to indicate compounds of the type MxHy and not necessarily to indicate that any compounds listed behave as hydrides chemically.

* none listed

Fluorides

* AuF3: gold (III) fluoride
* AuF5: gold (V) fluoride

Chlorides

* AuCl: gold (I) chloride
* [AuCl3]2: gold (III) chloride
* Au4Cl8: gold (I, III) chloride

Bromides

* AuBr: gold (I) bromide
* [AuBr3]2: gold (III) bromide

Iodides

* AuI: gold (I) iodide
* AuI3: gold (III) iodide

Oxides

* Au2O3: gold (III) oxide

Sulfides

* Au2S: gold (I) sulphide
* Au2S3: gold (III) sulphide

Selenides

* AuSe: gold (I, III) selenide
* Au2Se3: gold (III) selenide

Tellurides

* AuTe2: gold ditelluride

Nitrides

* none listed

Carbonyls

* none listed

Complexes

* none listed

Although the Egyptians knew of the metaphysical and healing powers of gold, it was the great alchemist Paracelsus who first prepared gold colloid solution in modern times. He called his purple solution of gold Aurum Potable and believed it cured all manner of physical, mental, and spiritual ailments. "Gold receives its influence from the Sun," he wrote, "which is, as it were, the Heart of the world and by communicating these influences to the human heart it serves to fortify and cleanse it from all impurities." The alchemists believed that gold represented the perfection of matter, and that its presence in the body would enliven, rejuvenate, and cure a multitude of disturbances in the life force balance of the body. In fact, the alchemists believed colloidal gold had a balancing and harmonizing effect on all levels of body, mind, and spirit. It was used to improve mental attitude and treat unstable mental and emotional states such as depression, melancholy, sorrow, fear, despair, anguish, frustration, suicidal tendencies, seasonal affective disorder, poor memory, poor concentration, and many other unbalances in mind, body, and spirit.

If metallic gold is divided into fine particles with sizes ranging from one to one hundred billionths of a meter, the particles are permanently suspended in solution (it becomes colloidal) and exhibits new properties due to the larger amount of gold surface area available. After studying the work of Paracelsus, the English scientist Michael Faraday prepared colloidal gold in 1857, and many uses were found for his solutions of "activated gold." In 1890, the distinguished German bacteriologist Robert Koch won the Nobel Prize for his discovery that compounds made with gold inhibited growth of bacteria.

The metal gold never corrodes or even tarnishes, is completely non-toxic, and exhibits no interactions with other drugs. Gold is the only heavy metal that has a right- hand atomic spin and is therefore easily tolerated by the body. The mystical metal has been used for both spiritual and medical purposes as far back as ancient Egypt. Over 5,000 years ago, the Egyptians used gold in dentistry and ingested it for mental, bodily, and spiritual purification. The ancients believed that gold in the body worked by stimulating the chi (life force) and raising the level of vibration on all levels. In Alexandria, alchemists developed a powerful colloidal elixir known as "liquid gold," which reportedly had the ability to restore youth.

In ancient Rome, gold salves were used for the treatment of disfiguring skin lesions and ulcers, and today, gold leaf plays an important role in the treatment of chronic skin ulcers. The great alchemist and founder of modern medicine, Paracelsus, developed many highly successful treatments from metallic minerals including gold. In medieval Europe, gold-coated pills and colloids ("gold waters") were extremely popular. Alchemists mixed powdered gold into drinks to "comfort sore limbs," and today, it is widely used in the treatment of rheumatoid arthritis. In the 1900s, surgeons actually implanted a $5 gold piece under the skin near an inflamed joint, such as a knee or elbow. In China, peasants still cook their rice with a gold coin in order to help replenish gold in their bodies, and fancy Chinese restaurants put 24-karat gold-leaf in their food preparations. Today, gold netting is used in surgery to patch damaged blood vessels, nerves, bones, and membranes. Modern physicians Inject microscopic gold to help retard prostate cancer in men and women with ovarian cancer are treated with gold solutions. Gold vapor lasers seek out and destroy cancerous cells without harming their healthy neighbors or give new life to patients with once inoperable heart conditions and tumors. One experimental new gold compound blocks virus replication in infected cells and is being tested for the treatment of AIDS. By attaching a molecular marker to a microscopic piece of gold, scientists can follow its movement through the body. Some researchers are placing gold on DNA to study the hybrid genetic material in cells, while others are using it to determine how cells respond to toxins, heat and physical stress. Because it is biologically benign and easy to trace, biochemists use gold to form compounds with proteins to create new lifesaving drugs. Gold is truly the perfection of the metals.

Making of Hyssop Stone

This would be used in plant alchemy or alchemy in laboratory (plant stones and essences) Everyone has their own methods of working but in the end when done with the separatory and purification parts of the alchemical work one should have at the very least 3 of the alchemical elements front of them. At minimum these would be the crystalline salts of the herb, its volatile essential oil -if the plant has any, and of course the alcohol obtained from the herb or wine via distillation.

The job of the alchemist is then to combine these three in such a way that a union begins to take place, and the salts which outwardly seem hard and impervious begin to drink up the liquid fractions introduced to them. Drop by drop these liquid fractions are added, until the salts begin to change their nature and appearance. Slowly they become darker in color ranging from pale amber, to a deep rusty red. The salts become sticky and adhere to one another.

The above takes time and patience a minimum we have found of 3 months to bring about this state, and yet it is not done. For Nature left to her devises has a surprise, for the artist a marriage much spoken of but seldom seen, the union of opposites, into a singular new divine child. It is only through art, assisting Nature that her subject can be brought to such an exalted state. In the dark warmth of the incubator the many become one, what was solid, now flows, what was obstructive to light, is now translucent. The work is now though just truly beginning for the nascent stone must be feed and tempered by the artist. Finally the red powder of projection is added and the final casting of the stone is made. Where before the gentle heat of one's own hand would have been enough to cause the stone to melt like wax, it now resist fluxing for it like the salamander has learned to love the flame. Do not think though that your stone can not flow for it can, as placing it in the oven at 200 F will bring about its fluxing but with no smoke. Too, if left out and exposed to the air, the stone will begin to run in time. We have heard people say that this should not be so, we refer them to "Collectanea Chemica" in which the Adept writes "You have, by carefully following our directions above, procured the tinctures, white or yellow, in the Vegetable Kingdom. The yellow is more efficacious if the work is well performed; either of them, by being exposed in the air, will soon run into a thick, essential oil, smelling very strong of the plant..."

Oils of Metals

We begin by taking raw metal ore and crushing it. Then the ore is calcined repeatedly at first its basic color remains. Slowly a red hue appears in the ore. But the ore is still as an uncooked meat and not fit for use in any alchemical work. The red hue grows more distinct and is a sign of the ore nearing completion. Finally the ore becomes a light grey and our work of calcination is almost done. When the ore reaches a light beige color to white is ready for the next stage of the work. Interestingly, metallic elixirs from both Eastern and Western alchemical approaches are prepared by methods strikingly different, and yet they create an oil which belies the inorganic quality of the source. Many oils by definition float on water and sink when in alcohol, containing heavy salt crystals that are in dissolution.

Medicinal Qualities of Metallic Oils

1) Gold Oil - The Sun

This oil is prepared from the ashes of gold (calcinated gold of 24K) which cannot return to the metallic state. Those ashes are fused into a colorful glass with special alchemical salts elaborated from a phosphoric principle.

Those highly fixed salts are then combined naturally with the universal spirit which contains corporified light or astral fire. When exposed several nights to the full moon, this glass dissolves by attraction into an oily thick paste. This oil which is the soul and heavier falls to the bottom; the spirit which is lighter floats on top. So, you have to shake the bottle before use.

This gold oil is excellent for leukemia patients as the highly fixed phosphoric principle will join by the law of affinity with its corresponding human phosphoric principle within the bones. Thus it will establish itself there and do its work of regeneration from within.

Silver Oil - The Moon

This oil is prepared from metallic ashes of silver which cannot return to the metallic state. Those ashes are fused into a colorful glass with special alchemical salts elaborated from a phosphoric principle. Those highly fixed salts are then combined naturally with the universal spirit which contains corporified light or astral fire. When exposed several nights to the full moon, this glass dissolves by attraction into an oily thick paste. The oil which is the soul and heavier falls to the bottom; the spirit which is lighter floats on top. So, you have to shake the bottle before use.

The moon, silver, rules the brain, the skin and the sexual organs in females. The silver oil is very useful for children suffering of night terrors and those children who "look old." It is good for female sterility, also for almost constitutional dysmenorrhoea if given in the first half of the menstrual cycle. It is also good for curing dry constipation. Excellent in controlling mental illnesses and chronic diseases of the brain.

2) Iron Oil (Black) - The Mars

This oil is made from an ore widely found in the Himalayan belt. This black sticky ore is first purified and made soluble. It is then distilled very slowly in a glass retort to release its thick oily soul (approximately 15 per cent of its weight).

It is excellent for: diabetes, male and female sterility, as a strong tonic it is highly recommended in general debility due to old age; bronchial disorders; asthma; piles, inflammation, digestive disorders like dyspepsia; worms, constipation; skin ailments; blood pressure and sexual impotency.

Note: The treatment should not exceed 40 days as it could increase blood pressure. It must not be given to kidney stone or gall-bladder stone patients.

3) Iron Oil (Red) - Mars

This oil is made from red magnetite ore, iron pyrites and iron ashes (incinerated iron) dissolved in a strong vegetable alkali alchemically prepared from oak wood. This metallic solution when put in a warm place for digestion starts to precipitate into an earth. This earth then ferments and swells thus releasing a gaseous vapor in the form of thousands of bubbles and foam. When the fermentation is completed, the matter has completely putrefied while passing through various colors which culminate in a pith-black tar-like substance. The body is then considered dead as it has released or given up its soul in the form of a fiery red oil.

Mars rules the gall-bladder and the larynx. So this oil is excellent for curing ailments related to these organs. Due to its power of fixation iron has a great anti-toxic function against several poisoning substances such as arsenic, lead, mercury, copper, and cyanide. It is also indispensable to fix and strengthen will power and consolidate the nervous system in cases of neurosis and convalescence.

4) Mercury Oil - Mercury

This oil is made from purified medicinal mercury which has been processed to absorb in itself the essence of copper. In Indian alchemy it is said that this mercury has received 5 impressions or memories. This mercury is alchemically joined to purified medicinal sulphur by the agency of a salt, thus becoming a bright red exalted alchemical cinnabar. On being exposed several nights to the full moon it resolves itself into a blood like oil by attracting the universal spirit of the world in the form of corporified light.

To this oil, essences of gold and mica are added along with pure musk, ambergris oil, Baltic Russian amber paste, saffron and gorochand, which is a rare orange stone-like animal substance.

Mercury rules the lungs, the lymphs and the nerves. It is very useful in paralysis, hemiplegia and several nervous disorders such as Zona. It is also a very helpful agent in treating certain cancers, especially of the lungs.

Ideal for young lymphatic children and the ones suffering of stagnation. It removes obsessions, fixed ideas, mental viscosity and deep depression of "lung type." In the light geriatrics, it is a powerful regenerator of the immune system, nervous system, if combined with several mineral essences such as gold, mica, etc, and a strong sexual tonic when animal essences such as musk or ambergris are added.

5) Copper Oil - Venus

This oil is made from a fine chalcopyrite found in a French mine. This ore contains an average of 10 grams of gold per ton. To this, ashes of incinerated copper are added. They are then dissolved in a strong vegetable alkali alchemically prepared from oak wood. This metallic solution when put in a warm place for digestion starts to precipitate into an earth. This earth then ferments and swells thus releasing a gaseous vapor in the form of thousands of bubbles and foam. When the fermentation is completed, the matter has completely putrefied while passing through various beautiful colors which culminate in a pitch-black, tar-like substance. The body is then considered dead as it has released or given up its soul in the form of a fiery red oil. This is called the solution or the separation of the elements.

Venus, or copper, rules the kidneys and the veins. It is very useful in controlling the bad effect of an excess of its metal in polarity: iron. It is a powerful antispasmodic. It stimulates the veinous stasi in the human organism, and it removes the affections of its key-organ the kidneys, and also the thyroid. It is excellent in post traumatic problems such as accident, surgery, and in convalescence. It removes body pain of rheumatic origin, inflammation, swelling, etc.

6) Tin Oil - Jupiter

This oil is made from ashes of incinerated tin, which cannot return to the metallic state. These ashes are then dissolved in a strong vegetable alkali alchemically prepared from oak wood. This metallic solution, when put in a warm place for digestion, starts to precipitate into an earth. This earth swells and ferments, thus releasing a gaseous vapor in the form of thousands of bubbles and foam. When the fermentation is completed, the matter has completely putrefied while passing through various beautiful soft colors which culminate in a black tar-like substance. The body is then considered dead as it has released or given up its soul in the form of a fiery orange oil. This is called the solution or the separation of the elements. Jupiter or Tin rules the liver, the cartilage and the muscles. This oil is excellent in case of someone "loosing shape." Its key organ is the liver; thus it is best for jaundice;

hepatitis; cirrhosis; certain types of eczema; liquid ovarian cysts; inflammatory effusions; pleurisies; certain phases of manic-depressive people; certain types of obesity. It is an excellent antidote for the bad effects of its metal in polarity: mercury.

7) Lead Oil (Saturn)

This oil is made from the ashes of incinerated lead and from good lead ore (Galena). These are then dissolved in a strong vegetable alkali alchemically prepared from oak wood. This metallic solution, when put in a warm place for digestion, starts to precipitate into an earth. This earth swells and ferments, thus releasing a gaseous vapor in the form of thousands of bubbles and foam. When the fermentation is completed, the matter has completely putrefied while passing through various colors, which culminate in a black tar-like substance. The body is then considered dead as it has released or given up its soul in the form of a fiery red oil. This is called the solution or the separation of the elements.

Saturn, or lead, rules the spleen, the skeleton, and the marrow. It is useful to control an excessive imagination, and also hallucinations due to neurological delirious after- effects. (encephalitis, post-traumatic troubles). It favors ossification and structuring. It is precious for osteoporosis and metastasis of the bones. It is also very useful for the spleen and its ailments. It is better not to take this oil in the period of the rising, full moon, to replace it with silver, which is its metal in polarity.

8) Antimony Oil

This oil is made from excellent stibnite (antimony ore) found in the French Britannia, and from an alchemically prepared antimony metal exalted with iron. These are then dissolved in a strong vegetable alkali alchemically prepared from oak wood. This metallic solution, when put in a warm place to digest, starts to precipitate into an earth. This earth swells and ferments, thus releasing a gaseous vapor in the form of thousands of bubbles and foam. When the fermentation is completed, the matter has completely putrefied while passing through various beautiful colors, which culminate in a black tar-like substance, The body is then considered dead as it has released or given up its soul in the form of a fiery red oil. This is called the solution or the separation of the elements.

Antimony is excellent for all ailments of the lungs and the bronchial tubes. It is good for asthma. It greatly favors expectoration and removes excess of phlegm from the lungs. It is very efficient for those who suffer from chronic breathing problems.

Dose: One drop in a 200ml bowl of hot instant soup, preferably in the morning once in a while or daily for acute or chronic cases.

9) Potable Gold - Sun

It is a liquor called by the ancient masters "Potable Gold." It is obtained by a divine process and it is made from the finest and purest seminal gold, which appears as a volatile red-brown greasy earth, which is then dissolved into a liquor. It is also called by the ancient "The universal medicine of the first order."

In the light of geriatrics, it is considered the king of medicines as it is endowed with extraordinary virtues to regenerate the human body and to cure most illnesses.

It is excellent for most cancers and also for the heart. It is also a powerful stimulant of the liver etc. It dissolves kidney-stones and the gall-bladder stones.

It can be added to ant vegetable medicinal extract in order to greatly amplify its virtues. It can also be added to metallic oils as well. It can be used in almost any emergency. When absorbed, it can generate a lot of heat in the body, thus provoking natural profuse sweating by which the impurities are expelled.

Dose: One drop a day for seven days in a glass of wine or in any drinks or in a cup of hot instant soup; then one drop a week in drinks only for a while.

11

Spagyrics: The Future in Medicine

"The world speaks to me in colors, my soul answers in music"

—Rabindranath Tagore (1861-1941)

Cells are composed of three basic parts, a nucleus, or brain of the cell, the cytoplasm, which provides nourishment to the cells nucleus, and the cell membrane, which contains both and gives it form and protection.

The cell is a chemical factory in which hundreds of chemical reactions take place. The "brain" or nucleus of the cell controls everything that goes on in this factory.

It is a necessary function of the cell membrane to let in proper nutrients to fuel this factory and keep out all harmful substances like bacteria and viruses.

Energy is produced through the burning of oxygen and sugar in the cell. The catalyst for this process is in the form of an enzyme. The enzyme gathers necessary raw material for the reactions to take place and acts as a catalyst for the reaction. Should that enzyme be lacking the exact sequence of reactions is not possible and the cell cannot survive.

The enzymes in a cell wear out after a while. The nucleus acts as a template to produce more enzymes. The enzymes must be constructed out of basic materials, namely proteins, vitamins, and minerals. If your diet is deficient in these ingredients then the cell cannot properly replenish the enzymes. The chemical factory comes to a halt and the cell dies.

You must get all the raw materials needed on a daily basis.

The cytoplasm contains all the basic salts. Different types of cells require more or less of certain of the salts for example nerve cells, require larger amounts of Kali Phosphate to function. Blood cells higher amounts of Ferrum phosphate.

Although proper nutrition of course is also important to the health of the body and cells, vitamin supplements and diet often overlook these essential micro nutrients salts that the cells need to remain healthy.

Cell enzymes work to attract the necessary raw materials by electrical attraction. The cells are the building blocks of the body. All our internal organs our skin our blood all made up of cells. The health of our body is dependent upon the health of the smallest part of our body; the cell.

Our cells are replaced cyclically on a regular basis. When the cell does not have the proper materials that it needs to be a healthy cell, our overall health suffers. Cell Salts provide the components that our cells need to be healthy. Taken on a regular basis over a period of time our cells rebuild themselves with the proper healthy materials that we need.

In 1873, German biochemist, William H. Schuessler found that there are certain essential minerals that the body requires. He discovered this by studying the remains of numerous cadavers and examining them after calcinations or burning to see what essential elements remained.

He found that an imbalance or a lack of any of these minerals may lead to disease in the tissues so lacking. Providing the missing minerals to the tissues corrects that imbalance and so eliminates the illness.

Thus the cell salts provide a rebalancing of the body enabling its natural disease controlling mechanisms to function. To this end, the cell salts are not a "cure" or a medicine per se but a body function balancing supplement albeit a powerful one nonetheless.

It was also found as well that the cell salts provide remedies for many illnesses, not as a medicine, but as an enhancer for the health of the body on a cell level, helping the body to heal itself.

The full spectrum salts, *viz.* minerals and trace elements, provides effective amounts of magnesium, sodium, chlorine, and lithium, which are essential to have a wonderful balancing effect on the immune system.

Due to a lack of trace elements in the soil, even in most 'organically' farmed soils, trace element deficiency in modern society is almost universal. This is true even if you eat a healthy diet with plenty of organic food grains, fruits and vegetables, include raw vegetable juices in your diet or consume trace element rich supplements, it been repeatedly found that the major trace elements of Selenium, Zinc, Chromium, Iron, Manganese, Boron, etc. are required in certain quantities to optimise health. We each have, for inherited, constitutional and lifestyle reasons, special needs for a certain quantity of trace elements to achieve full health, and in many cases, to be disease free.

Trace elements are involved in enzymatic activities, immunological reactions, physiological mechanisms and carcinogenesis. Deficiency in some trace elements, such as iron and iodine, is still an important health problem, especially in developing countries. Some groups of individuals are more likely to develop trace element deficiency. The role of trace elements deficiency is suspected in various clinical situations and is now confirmed by well designed supplementation studies. Although toxicity of trace elements with clinical manifestations is rare, it has been observed that manganese toxicity may occur in patients receiving parenteral nutrition. Recent data about trace elements deficiency and toxicity are indicated in this review.

Advances in trace element research over the last decade have done much to elucidate the function of these nutrients at the biochemical level. Five new trace elements have been identified and the general relevance of microelements in human nutrition has undergone reassessment. Deficiencies of iodine, iron and fluorine remain important problems and necessitate supplementation. Suboptimal nutrition in chromium, copper, selenium, zinc and possibly vanadium has been suggested, and these elements are generally acknowledged to be of concern in human nutrition. Genetic factors and other "conditioning" agents have been implicated in the aetiology of a number of trace element deficiencies in apparently well nourished communities. Tissues under anabolic stress have been recognized to be especially sensitive to trace element deficits, and the particular vulnerability of the fetus has been demonstrated on a number of occasions. In practical dietary terms, the loss of microelements during the refining and processing of food has been widely illustrated. Also, the generally lower levels of trace elements in plant material and the lower availability of minerals from these food sources has been well established. Of the newer trace element deficiencies, zinc impoverishment appears to be especially important, as a state of physiological zinc deficiency rapidly follows dietary insufficiency, and the consequences on all growing tissues are particularly serious. In general, recent developments suggest that marginal deficiencies of microelements are more widespread in human nutrition than was previously appreciated. Greater attention to trace element status seems to be indicated in circumstances in which physical condition and vigour are unaccountably poor and especially in situations accompanied by active anabolism.

As opined by Karen Bartlett the cell salts have serious characteristics in conjunction with the unique process known as spagyrics and it's role in human therapeutics.

Cell salts are homeopathic preparations of certain mineral compounds found within all living things. Cell salts represent a self contained homeopathic system that lends itself to easy home use. These trace elements are essential for the health and growth of the body. They are grouped in fours; Phosphates, Chlorides, Sulphates, and Fluorides (also Silica).This system of Medicine is based upon the "cell theory" of Virchow in 1858. He said that the body is a collection of cells and that all medical treatment should center around the health of the individual cell. Together with Schuessler, they developed a system of medicine based on cellular health.

Thus the cell salts provide a rebalancing of the body enabling its natural disease controlling mechanisms to function. To this end, the cell salts are not a "cure" or a medicine per se but a body function balancing supplement albeit a powerful one nonetheless.

The importance of the inorganic components of cells were recognized, hence the trace elements are found to be the basic building blocks of the cell and water and other organic substances were used by the salts in building the cells of the body.

Charles W. Littlefield, analytical chemist, wrote: "the mineral salts are, in a very real sense, the material basis of the organs and tissues of the body and are absolutely essential to their integrity of structure and functional activity. Experiments prove that the various tissue salts will rapidly disintegrate in the absence of the proper proportion of these salts in the circulation fluid. Whereas the maintenance of this proportion insures healthy growth and perpetual renewal.

These mineral salts are, therefore, the physical basis of all healing. Regardless of the school employed, if these are absent from the blood and tissues, no permanent cure is possible."

As reported by Nielsen F H of US Department of Agriculture, Grand Forks Human Nutrition Research Center, ND 58202 "the possible importance of some new essential trace elements in nutrition is discussed. Most likely, insufficient intake of a specific trace element becomes obvious only when the body is stressed in some way that enhances the need for that element; this has been supported by recent findings with selenium. The trace elements boron and copper may be of nutritional significance in a manner similar to selenium. When the diets of animals and humans are manipulated to cause possible changes in cellular integrity or in hormone responsiveness, a large number of responses to dietary boron occur. The findings indicate that boron is important for optimal calcium and, thus, bone metabolism. High dietary cystine and fructose exacerbate the signs of copper deficiency in rats; this indicates that the response to copper deficiency by humans would vary with the amino acid and carbohydrate composition of the diet. There is some evidence that chromium, molybdenum, nickel, arsenic, and vanadium may also be of nutritional significance under stress conditions. In other words, an increasing number of studies have been performed that have examined the importance of trace element nutritive in various forms of nutritional, metabolic, hormonal, or physiologic stress in animals and humans. These studies indicate that situations will be found in which a trace element is of nutritional significance. It is likely that some of the trace elements are more important in human nutrition than is now generally acknowledged."

Due to the minute scale of cells, the ideal way to replenish any deficiency is through very small micronutrients that go directly to the depleted cells.

Tinctures of the salts provide an easily absorbed transport for the body, enabling the needed salts to go directly to the bloodstream without the body expending much needed energy in digesting and processing the micronutrient cell salts.

According to Robert Bartlett Our cells are replaced cyclically on a regular basis. When the cell does not have the proper materials that it needs to be a healthy cell, our overall health suffers. Cell Salts provide the components that our cells need to be healthy. Taken on a regular basis over a period of time our cells rebuild themselves with the proper healthy materials that we need. All our internal organs our skin our blood all made up of cells. The health of our body is dependent upon the health of the smallest part of our body; the cell. These Salt level extracts contain the spagyric essence, which is made by purifying the plant or mineral body until it becomes a clear or white crystalline salt, and then adding the salt to the alcohol tincture to capture the physical signatures of the plant or mineral. This part of the extract serves to give the essence "body" in alchemical terms and helps to carry its healing actions into the physical.

According to Kristine Danowski, ancient Alchemy combined both the practical and the mystical. Practical chemistry included metallurgy (mining and purification of metals for weaponry, jewelry, and coins), art (paints, inks, dyes), medicine (various healing herbs and herbal preparations, funeral rites), and the mundane (flavoring herbs, spices, cosmetics). For example, ancient texts describe metallurgical methods that, when followed as written, produce quantitative yields of nearly pure metals. Civilizations depended on these metals, so naturally they would know how to extract and purify them. Mystical chemistry was the search for the Philosopher's Stone, symbolism, and various theories about the origin of matter.

That's where the Spagyric Medicine comes in.

A spagyric tincture is made by a careful process in which all the parts of the mineral or plant that you are working with is separated through a process of heat and distillation and each part is brought to it's highest and purest potential state. And so you essentially separate it into Mind, Body, and Spirit and as Alchemy assumes, each mineral and plant has each of these.

Having brought them to their highest evolutionary state (essentially speeding up the evolution through this method) the Parts are then recombined, giving you a superior "living tincture".

As all the "bodies" of each part of the mineral or plant have been separated and perfected, when they are recombined and brought into the body, the effect carries over to the person taking the remedy. Thus affecting a cure not only on the physical but also on the subtle level's of the body as well.

As we all have an Energy Body as well as a Physical Body. These tinctures then resonate with that Chi flow in the Body. And it is well documented that this is an important part of healing as proved in the results shown by Acupuncture, Acupressure, Therapeutic Touch, and many other systems that work on the subtle energy bodies of both humans and animals

It is this that makes a spagyric tincture superior and what makes the medicine unique. Right down to the actual mother salts prepared in this manner. The salts themselves were mined from the earth, carefully prepared in a year long process and aged like fine wines.

Some thirty elements, more or less, have been ascertained by different investigators as appearing in the human body. It has been definitely established that many of these are absolutely essential to physical construction. Iodine, number 53 of the elements, is regarded as the highest in atomic weight; and as we have pointed out, only the three that we have questioned appear in the antipsoric list beyond iodine.

The following list of elements appearing in the human body has been compiled from several sources. It is notable that not all these elements have been assigned constructive roles, in the eyes of investigators; or rather, their presence in the body structure has not been determined. Nevertheless, all these come within the first fifty-three elements, as determined by atomic weight.

1. Hydrogen
3. Lithium
6. Carbon
7. Nitrogen
8. Oxygen
9. Fluorine
11. Sodium
12. Magnesium
13. Aluminium
14. Silicon
15. Phosphorus
16. Sulphur
17. Chlorine
19. Potassium
20. Calcium
22. Titanium
25. Manganese
26. Iron
27. Cobalt
28. Nickel
29. Copper
30. Zinc
32. Germanium
33. Arsenic
35. Bromine
50. Tin
53. Iodine

The body elements best known to the student of biochemistry are: Hydrogen, Oxygen, Carbon, Nitrogen, Fluorine, Sodium, Magnesium, Silicon, Phosphorus, Sulphur, Chlorine, Potassium,

Calcium, Manganese, Iron, Copper, Zinc, Arsenic and Iodine. Chemists have been able to estimate the percentage of these elements present in the organism, even such small amounts as those of arsenic, with its sixth-decimal proportions in thyroid and brain, and 0.000,001,9 per cent. in the liver. It is comparatively easy to define the constructive purposes of many of these elements, such as calcium; yet there is some purpose aside from that of mere bricks-and-mortar for even the most obvious. Magnesium is found throughout the body, in the lungs, glands, brain, muscles and muscular organs such as the heart. This has been determined with a fair amount of measurable accuracy; yet how do we account for the fact that a magnesium-free diet sends animals into convulsions? Or that tin, found in traces in the tongue and brain, is related definitely to the sense of taste? When cobalt and nickel, discovered in the pancreas, are lacking, just what influence does this have in the development of diabetes?

Manganese is an accompaniment of iron in practically all human tissue. Scientists have discovered that manganese starvation in animals will produce sterility in the male and loss of mother-love in the female; this loss of maternal instinct incites them to refuse attention to their young, who die in a few hours. McCollum tells us: "*When to the carefully prepared manganese-free diet is added as little as five-thousandths of one per cent. of manganese, all the abnormalities described are corrected.*" Yet Reiman and Minot tell us: "*Prolonged feeding of moderate amounts of its ores to dogs failed to produce significant changes in the manganese content of the blood and tissues or to cause any pathological symptoms.*"

It is comparatively easy to determine the broader outlines of the constructive duties of these elements and inorganic substances, but it is the subtle and potential influences (as illustrated by the observations on manganese) that are most pertinent to our thesis. In other words, it is not the overfeeding or gross starvation of any element that provides us with the so-called antipsoric remedies. Since the so-called psoric conditions are largely functional and react preeminently upon the nervous and emotional plane, may we not regard these conditions as a lack of balance in the ability to assimilate, as well as a possible starvation of essentials?

In a comparison of the constructive role of these substances (as determined by laboratory technique) with their more subtle manifestations (demonstrated through provings of the homoeopathic potentiations), let us look again at manganese:

Reiman and Minot (J. Biological Chemistry) "found it to be present in practically all human tissue, the liver carrying more than any other;" J. H. Clarke (Dictionary of the Materia Medica) cites its ability to produce inflammation and fatty degeneration of the liver. We have seen its association with iron in the blood, and homoeopathically, it has its place in anemic conditions when indicated. We have noted the laboratory observation of the loss of maternal instinct. Clarke gives as the first mental symptom: "*Peevishness and taciturnity, with concentration in self.*" Sterility has not been a proven symptom, yet Clarke gives: "*Sensation of weakness in (male) genital organs.*"

Speaking of the necessity for carbohydrates in the diet, McCollum (Food, Nutrition and Health) says: "*During digestion and absorption through the intestinal walls all of these (forms of carbohydrates) are converted into glucose. Glucose is the one sugar which always occurs in the blood. Although it is present in blood only to the extent of one part per thousand of blood, this sugar is the principal fuel which is burned by the muscles for providing energy for keeping the body warm and for muscular work.*"

A cell possesses two characteristics, capacitance and inductance, which are the elements of a tuned circuit like a radio. Nano particles of high energy iridium and rhodium and iridium function so similarly that they are often called twins. Rhodium and iridium assist in the efficiency and performance of the neural circuitry, in the synaptic connections. Using these increases clarity and discerning power of the brain. It is estimated that over 6 per cent of the brain tissue by dry matter weight, is Rhodium and Iridium. 5 per cent of our nervous system is composed of monatomic elements.

During heightened activation the body can transmute certain palladium group elements such as Iridium and Rhodium into their high spin state by adding energy in the form of photons to the atoms.

It is through this high spin atomic nervous system that we achieve cosmic consciousness, the Philosopher's mind and ESP and spiritual phenomena Kundalini has the effect of stimulating an increased flow of ions upping the body's dipole and increasing the EMF. According to Siddha alchemical medicine literatures, mercury, iridium and rhodium have potent anti-aging properties.

Nowadays modern physics is affectionate with iridium, as in high spin it has been shown to have antigravity capabilities, and have been tried out in levitation experiments. The Kundalini ascent and descent can be assisted by Palladium group metals. Rhodium serves as the downflow of energy around the spinal column, iridium serves us the upflow. When these two are in balance, there is maximum coherence of these two energy currents. The two serpents coiled around a staff and surmounted by wings as the caduceus, the symbol of Western medicine seems inspired from Kundalini. Nano particle crystals which are not only bio absorbable, but are bonded with hydrogen to carry out specific electrical instructions in the body, including the activation of inert DNA. Considering you have 97 per cent junk DNA and the naturally obtained 12 strand DNA is now reduced to 2 strand DNA, you may find the role of DNA mutation in disease conditions.

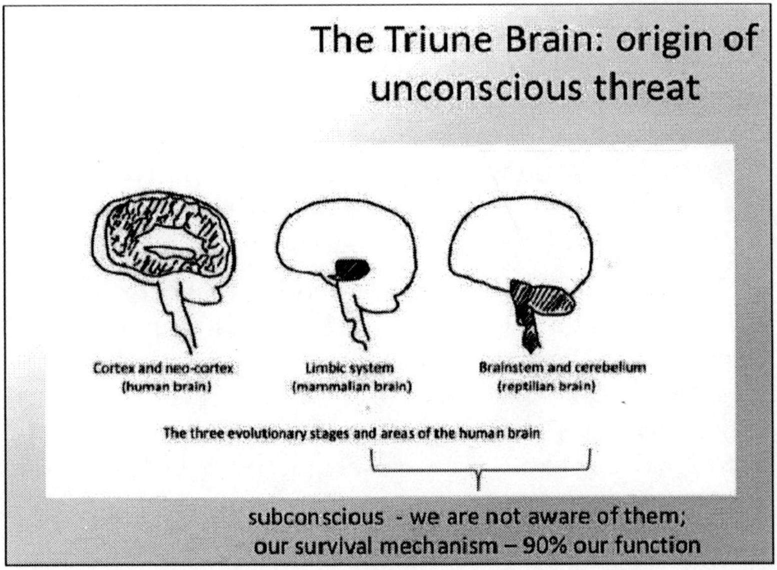

In 1992, Bruce Taino of Taino Technology, an independent division of Eastern State University in Cheny, Washington, built the first frequency monitor in the world. Taino has determined that the average frequency of a healthy human body during the day time is 62 to 68 Hz. When the frequency drops, the immune system is compromised. If the frequency drops to 58 Hz, cold and flu symptoms appear; at 55 Hz, diseases like Candida take hold; at 52 Hz, Epstein Bar and at 42 Hz, Cancer.

Dr. G. Young and Bruce Tainio also discovered that a healthy body from head to foot has a frequency ranging from 62-71 Hz during the day. When measuring the human body, it has been observed that a healthy human resonates at and above 59 to 62Hz. This measurement is taken at the abdominal level. The sternum to the upper throat area resonates at about 62-68 Hz. The entire head of a normal healthy human resonates at between 72-78 Hz., and this measurement may go as high as 90 Hz. during times of extreme mental activity. Disease begins at 58Hz., and becomes more severe at lower measurements, *i.e.*, cancer has a frequency of 42 Hz.6 It was also discovered that headaches are caused by a disturbance in the electrical fields between the right and left lobes of the brain. If the frequency varies by more than 3 Hz. headaches develop. If the frequency varies by more than 10 Hz. substantial or migraine-type headaches develop. It has been found that the normal healthy range of the human body is 62-68 Hertz. At this level and above, nobody had any ailments at all. Disease starts at: 58 MHz, Amongst other diseases, Colds and Flu start at: 57-60 MHz, Candida overgrowth starts at: 55 MHz, Receptive to Epstein Barr at: 52 MHz, Receptive to Cancer at: 42 MHz and Death occurs at: 25 MHz.

Everyone who had a common cold had a cellular frequency of 58Hz or less; for flu it was 57 Hz or less; candida symptoms began to appear at 55 Hz, for Epstein Barr virus it was 52 Hz. Everyone he measured who had some form of cancer had a cellular frequency of 42 Hz or less. Clearly, high frequency cells correspond with better health and ideally everyone should strive for a frequency of at least 62 Hz.

The biochemist and Nobel Prize winner Albert Lehninger of Johns Hopkins mentions that some reactions in the living cell happen quite a lot faster than what corresponds to 37C temperature. The explanation seems to be that the body purposely directs chemical reactions by means of electromagnetic vibrations (biophotons). Photons switch on the body's processes like an orchestra conductor bringing each individual instrument into the collective sound. At different frequencies, they perform different functions. Popp found that molecules in the cells responded to certain frequencies, and that a range of vibrations from the photons caused a variety of frequencies in other molecules of the body.

What has been proposed is that somehow each molecule sends out a unique electromagnetic field that can "sense" the field of the complimentary molecule. It's as if there is a "dance" in the cellular medium and the molecules move to the rhythm. The music is supplied by the biophoton.

Dr. Leonard Horowitz has opined that DNA emits and receives phonons and photons, the electromagnetic waves of sound and light.

As well, three Nobel laureates in medical research have asserted that the primary function of DNA is not to synthesize proteins, but to perform bioacoustic and bioelectrical signalling.

While research such as that by Fritz-Albert Popp shows that DNA is a biophoton emitter, other research suggests that sound actually originates light. These 'biophoton emission', as Popp called them, provided an ideal communication system for the transfer of information to many cells across the organism. Popp opined that quanta of light can initiate. or arrest, cascade-like reactions in the cells. and that genetic cellular damage can be virtually repaired within hours, by faint beams of light.

He further says, "*We are still on the threshold only understanding the complex relationship between light and life, but we can now say emphatically, that the function of our entire metabolism is dependent on light.*"

Biophotonics is a branch of quantum biology dealing with interactions between single- photons and biological matter in order to understand the inner workings of cells and tissues in living organisms. It is probably the best solution for understanding cell function by integrating molecular activities within the living cells. The term biophotons refers to coherent photons emitted from biological organisms, Biophoton theory concerns DNA as the most probable source of biophoton emission.Popp considered it to be a quantum biological phenomenon with bio-informational character distinct from the non-coherent emission of photons as by-products of metabolism, like thermal radiation and bioluminescence/ chemiluminescence caused by radical reactions, oxidation etc.

Biophoton emission originates from relaxation of electronically excited states of the constituents of living cells, which are generally associated with the presence of an oxidative metabolism that accompanies the production of reactive oxygen species which participate in the regulation of a wide spectrum of biochemical and physiological functions. This occurs in the visible and UV part of the electromagnetic spectrum at ultra low intensities, on the order of 10-16 - 10-18 w/cm2.

The coherent emission of bio-photons is connected to energy and information transfer processes in the biological organisms, and has been linked to the function of DNA and to gene regulation.

When we get a cut or scratch on our skin, the cells that are injured transmit signal the surrounding healthy cells to begin reproducing copies of themselves to fill in and mend the opening. When the skin is back to normal, a signal is sent to the cells to tell them to stop reproducing. Scientists have wondered exactly how this works.

This phenomenon of coordination and communication could only occur in a holistic system with one central orchestrator. Popp showed in his experiments that these weak light emissions were sufficient to orchestrate the body's repairs. The emissions had to be low intensity because these communications took place on a very small, intracellular, quantum level.

The Penrose–Hameroff theory of orchestrated objective reduction (Orch OR) claims that quantum computations in the brain account for consciousness.

The communication among neurons by the secretion of neurotransmitters is based on synaptic vesicles distributed along their axons. The neuronal cytoskeleton has a key role in the dynamics of these vesicles. In the 1990s, Stuart Hameroff, psychologist at the University of Arizona, Tucson, USA, and Roger Penrose, mathematical physicist at the University of Oxford, Oxford, UK, proposed that microtubules, the smallest units of the cytoskeleton, are channels for the transfer of the integrated quantum information responsible for consciousness.

In their paper, Hameroff and Penrose present a model linking microtubules to consciousness using quantum theory. In their model, quantum coherence emerges, and is isolated in brain microtubules until a threshold related to quantum gravity is reached. The resultant self-collapse creates an instantaneous "now" event. Sequences of such events create a flow of time, and consciousness.

It shows that the existence of internal photons—inner light—is very real and is the basis of virtually all human cellular and systemic function.

In a paper entitled "A Holographic Concept of Reality" by Richard Alan Miller, Burt Webb and Darden Dickson, of Department of Paraphysics and Parapsychology, Experimental College, University of Washington showed that superposed coherent waves in the cells interact and form patterns first through sound, and secondly through light.

Russian scientists Peter Gariaev and Vladimir Poponin demonstrated that chromosomes work like holographic biocomputers, using the DNA's own electromagnetic radiation to generate and interpret spiralling waves of sound and light that run up and down the DNA ladder. Gariaev and his group used language frequencies such as words (which are sounds) to repair chromosomes damaged by X-rays.

Gariaev thus concludes that life is electromagnetic rather than chemical and that DNA can be activated with linguistic expressions or sounds like an antenna. In turn, this activation modifies the human bioenergy fields, which transmit radio and light waves to bodily structures.

"When we activate the power of our hearts' commitment and intentionally have sincere feelings such as appreciation, care and love, we allow our hearts'

electrical energy to work for us. Consciously choosing a core heart feeling over a negative one means instead of the drain and damage stress causes to our bodies' systems, we are renewed mentally, physically and emotionally. The more we do this the better we're able to ward off stress and energy drains in the future. Positive feelings fortify our energy systems and nourish the body at the cellular level. We call these emotions quantum nutrients."

In simple terms most people can relate to, what this means is that when we are having a bad day, going through a rough period such as dealing with the sickness of a loved one or coping with financial troubles, we can actually influence our bodies; all the way down to the cellular level; by intentionally thinking positive thoughts and focusing on positive emotions.

DNA Regulation

When we are born, the deoxyribonucleic acid or DNA in our bodies contains the blueprints for who we are and instructions for who we will become. For example, it can tell our eyes to eventually turn from blue at birth to hazel later on, our length to grow from 20 inches to 70 and direct a multitude of other changes over the course of our lives.

Many people have mistakenly believed that the DNA with which we are born is the sole determinant for who we are and will become, but scientists have understood for decades that this genetic determinism is a flawed theory.

The field of epigenetics refers to the science that studies how the development, functioning and evolution of biological systems are influenced by forces operating outside the DNA sequence, including intracellular, environmental and energetic influences.

Researchers have shown through studies that epigenetics entails even more than DNA and the places where we live, the climate around us and all the twists, turns and hard knocks of our lives.

Stem cell biologist and bestselling author Bruce Lipton, Ph.D., says the distinction between genetic determinism and epigenetics is important.

"The difference between these two is significant because this fundamental belief called genetic determinism literally means that our lives, which are defined as our physical, physiological and emotional behavioral traits, are

controlled by the genetic code," Lipton said in an interview with the online magazine, Superconsciousness. *"This kind of belief system provides a visual picture of people being victims: If the genes control our life function, then our lives are being controlled by things outside of our ability to change them. This leads to victimization that the illnesses and diseases that run in families are propagated through the passing of genes associated with those attributes. Laboratory evidence shows this is not true."*

Quantum Nutrients

"When we have negative emotions such as anger, anxiety and dislike or hate, or exposed to negative thoughts or environment, we experience stress and our energy reserves are redirected," which causes a portion of our energy reserves, which otherwise would be put to work maintaining, repairing and regenerating our complex biological systems, to instead confront the stresses these negative thoughts and feelings create. Researchers opined that physical aspects of DNA strands could be influenced by human intention.

"The results provide experimental evidence to support the hypothesis that aspects of the DNA molecule can be altered through intentionality," the article states. "The data indicate that when individuals are in a heart-focused, loving state and in a more coherent mode of physiological functioning, they have a greater ability to alter the conformation of DNA. (Rollin McCraty, Mike Atkinson, and Dana Tomasino, "Modulation of DNA Conformation by Heart-Focused Intention" (publication no. 03-008, Boulder Creek, CA: Institute of HeartMath, 2003).

According to Doc Childre's theory of heart intelligence, the influence or control individuals can have on their DNA is linked through "*an energetic connection or coupling of information*" which occurs between the DNA in cells and higher dimensional structures the higher self or spirit.

Childre further postulates, the heart, which generates a much stronger electromagnetic field than the brain's, provides the energetic field that binds together the higher dimensional structures and the body's many systems as well as its DNA.

Spagyrics are rich in colloids which have several benefits to one on the spiritual path. Improved memory, higher conductivity, rejuvenation of cancerous cells, nerve stimulation and increased longevity are just a few scientifically proven effects of administering colloids to the body.

Indian Siddha and Ayurvedic medicine (4000 BC) have used rare elements like Gold, Iridium, and Platinum besides Silver and Mercury in therapeutics.

Gold eradicates pathogens reducing their ability to effect your immunity. Colloidal Gold improves the electrical signals in the nerve cells of the brain while also reducing swelling in conditions such as arthritis, bursitis, rheumatism, and tendinitis.

Iridium has been dubbed "the nutrient of consciousness" as Iridium is known to spark the biological reality of the ascension process. Key to transmission and reception.

Etymologically its name is connected to "a messenger" as it is often associated with the particles of space dust. It functions as a channel to resonate knowledge contained within such particles.

Platinum has a specialty in tissue regeneration for those who engage in rigorous workouts that often take the body to its limits. Gaining apex physical health can be obtained by going straight for the Platinum when mineralizing for any intense training. Platinum also promotes increased libido in both males and females.

Rarified atoms of gold suspended in water significantly change consciousness, both in perception, and processing ability - especially communication between both hemispheres. It is clinically proven to have a significant effect on depression, and in severe inflammatory conditions. It is used to suspend inefficient immune systems, to halt the progress of certain types of cancer and HIV. Leading research indicates that gold and platinum repair damaged DNA sequences. To restore health and end the vicious disease cycle, a medication must address all areas of dysfunction, on all levels of the human body. These 3 levels, when corrected simultaneously, provide the key to disrupting the pathophysiological cycle of illness and ensuring long-lasting health. This is the modern-day, scientific understanding of Body, Mind, and Spirit.

Biochemical–The Body

Biochemical Symptomatic Therapeutics

Western medicine works on the biochemical level. Treatment of pathological dysfunctions and regulation of biochemical actions in the body unfold at this stage, and the primary concern is to provide symptomatic relief.

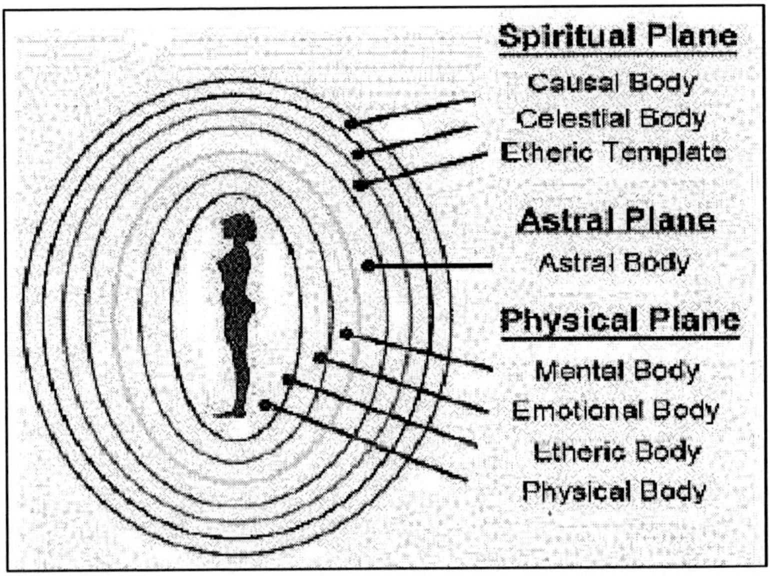

PNEI–The Mind

Psycho-Neuro-Endocrine-Immunological Regulation – Often referred to as Body- Mind medicine, this level is guided by emotions and the interaction between psychological processes and the nervous, neuro-immuno-endocrine system of the human body. PNEI studies, among other things, the physiological functioning of the neuroimmune system in health and disease; disorders of these systems (autoimmune diseases/hypersensitivities/ immune deficiency); and the physical, chemical and physiological characteristics of the PNEI related systems.

Informational–The Spirit

The Spiritual or informational quantum state level is responsible for bodily responses acting upon external and internal informational interchanges which adversely affect functioning on a cellular to a systematic level, and contribute to the formation of pathological dysfunction seen in the top level of the biochemical as disease. DNA science and genetics has proven features within DNA provide wave interchanges at this informational level that then interact with body's genetic material and exhibit into physical reactions that sustain life.

Any medical treatment that does not address all three levels of being falls short of truly restoring health. Western conventional medicine is focused on the physical body– the precise biochemical processes that cause physical symptoms.

Spagyric medicines provide a treatment of pathological dysfunctions and regulation of biochemical actions in the body. These sophisticated biological medications act on the biochemical level of the body and take into consideration pharmacological effects and actions on the physical body.

Psycho-Neuro-Endocrine-Immunology Regulation

Growing research in the field of Psycho-Neuro-Immunology (PNI) as well as the expanded field of Psycho-Neuro-Endocrine-Immunology (PNEI) over the last 30 years has shown how tightly coupled the mind and body are. There is now a huge body of published evidence documenting at the neurological and biochemical level, how states of mind such as anxiety, depression and anger affect the functioning of immune cells – T-cells, B-cells, Natural Killer cells, and macrophages. Effective regulation of the neuroendocrine balance is essential in the treatment of illness and has a profound impact on physiological responses and bioregulatory activity.

Spagyric influence on psycho-emotional level come through the special distillation process, which provides the distinctive fine-matter potentized homeopathic information that influence the psycho-emotional state of a patient. Spagyric medicine acts upon the various regulation mechanisms which comprise the psycho-neuro-endocrine-immune system and are connected to each other based on emotions which influence limbic activity, then hypothalamus and pituitary gland, and finally the sexual organs and adrenal glands. According to immune specialists, such as renowned immunologist Dr. Peter Schleicher, all levels of this PNEI hierarchy can be given regulatory impulses through the help of high quality spagyric medicines.

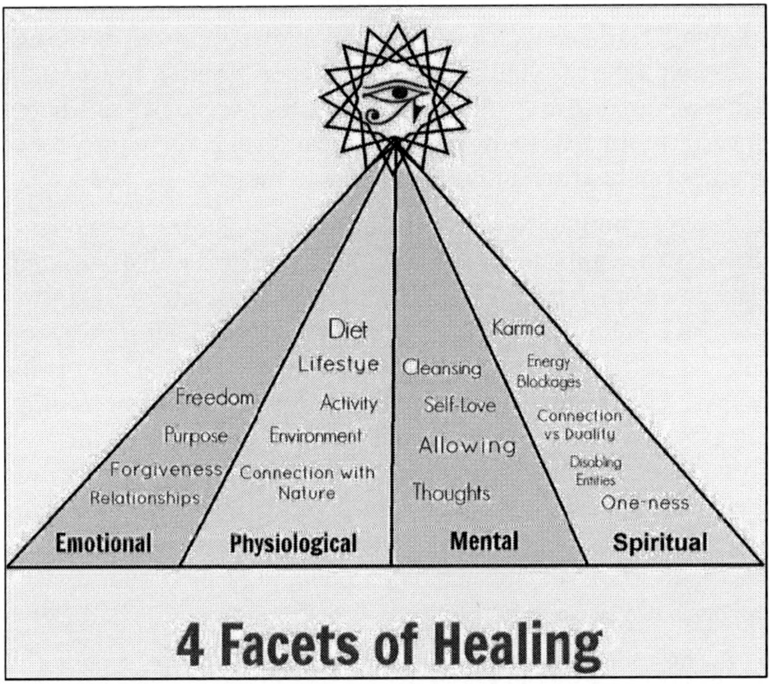

"*Ask anybody what the universe is made of, and you are likely told matter and energy. Yet, if we have learned anything from engineering, biology, and physics, information is just as crucial an ingredient.*"

– Physicist Jacob D. Bekenstein

The vast discoveries within quantum physics, that include but are not limited to quantum coherence, quantum entanglement, wave theory, and quantum information science, provide us an understanding of the importance information on the most basic quantum level has on the physical matter state of being. The study and progress in DNA science and genetics, such as Dr. Peter Gariaev's work in wave genetics, has proven features within DNA provide wave interchanges with the body's genetic information and this then exhibits into physical reactions that sustain life. So to do external informational interchanges with DNA and the body adversely affect functioning on a cellular to a systematic level, and contribute to the formation of pathological dysfunction seen in the top level of the physical as disease.

At this time scientific experiments at the Atomic Institute in Vienna demonstrate that different plants contain different radiation patterns (informational transfer signals). Every plant possesses a quite individual field of radiation: a particular 'energy fingerprint' that when provided to the human body in the proper manner can instruct and regulate functioning.

Spagyric influence on the quantum state informational level through the unification and enhancement of the distillate and macerate plant, herb, and mineral material. Utilizing the quantum state level information found in every biological substance, and enhancing its footprint through spagyric processing allows for deep level activation and regulation of cellular functioning. Spagyric medicines penetrate at this quantum level through hormones, chemicals, neurotransmitters, proteins, etc. and deliver the correct information to activate self-regulation of bodily systems and mechanisms. The reaction to this information then influences the higher states of emotional and physical health, and provides the basis of self-sustainable health.

In the book by Richard Hewitt '*The Quest To Regain Paradise*' the author demonstrated the true nature of the esoteric mysteries. Basically, the author suggests that all the different strands of the hermetic mysteries, Freemasonry, Rosicrucianism, Alchemy, Tarot, Astronomy, Magic etc, etc are all derived from a Hermetic source that was rendered into our DNA; moreover, that a message regarding this source – the details of a quest – can be decoded from our DNA.

Luc Montagnier discovered in 1982 the HIV virus and got the Nobel Prize in Medicine 2008, found that if a vial with DNA is diluted to a potency of at least D7 and then radiated with a low energy and very low electromagnetic frequency of 7 Hz – water in another vial that is within the same EMF field is changed in some way that after about 16 hours the vial with pure water contains some information of the source vial.

This information could be traced in 2 ways either by again radiating this target vial with 7 Hz and then measuring the resulting EMF spectrum or even more surprising by subjecting it to a Polymerase chain reaction process PCR that is otherwise used to make copies of DNA. The DNA created via this PCR process, in this vial of pure water, was almost identical than the original one.

Even more unexpectedly – both the process of sending DNA information as well as the reconstruction of the signal in the target vial only worked for dilutions equal or higher than D7.

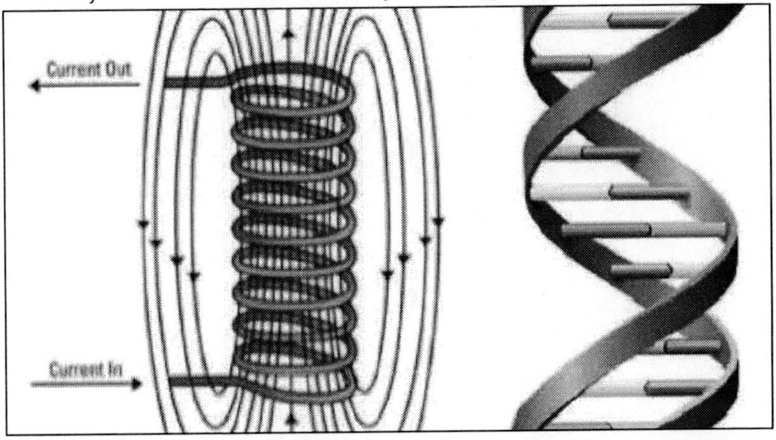

DNA Information Transfer via Electromagnetic Radiation (Luc Montagnier)

There are strong indications that EMF imprints information into water and this information is not destroyed but actually enhanced by vortex agitation and high dilution.

It is noteworthy that all these experiments were done with DNA and DNA has a coil structure like electric transformers. A coil structure is the physical means to create from an alternating electric current a magnetic field that is proportional to the number of windings of the coil. Also the other way round DNA could be possible also the receiver coils in our body to transform ambient magnetic fields into electric energy that powers as well as controls our cells.

Part 2

12

Pharmacy in Plant Alchemy

The word pharmacy is derived from the greek word "pharmakon', which means combining from denoting relationship to drug or medicine. It is a process of preparing the drugs, which includes sophistication in raw material analysis, analysis of chemical components, methods of preservation, combination and standardisation of drugs, also, art of compounding and dispensing them.

The synonym of the word Pharmacist is 'Apothecaries'. The term Pharmaceuticals refers to the physical chemistry of drugs and clinical pharmacy. Herbal Alchemy deals in particular art of preparation, preservation, combining and compounding the medicines.

The roots of modern pharmacy are in Alchemy. What is Alchemy? it seems appropriate to ponder on what Alchemy might be and how this pondering can lead us to spiritual progress. At this point, it is perhaps easier to describe what alchemy is not, rather than what it is. From a material point of view, Alchemy is neither chemistry nor hyperchemistry, but a biodynamic process more closely related to fermentation or putrefaction than to classical chemical reactions. Alchemy leads to a profound knowledge of the fundamental mechanisms of nature, yet is contrary to profane science which only considers the material aspects of these mechanisms. Alchemy considers the spiritual aspect as well as which is generally invisible to the sensory perception of the operator. This aspect of alchemical study brings the operator to spiritual progress, to a higher level of consciousness. The duality of this method of spiritual advancement has a great advantage over other methods. Spiritual advancement "makes one high" but, in order to accomplish the work, the Alchemist must remain grounded. He becomes aware of higher realities while he keeps in mind the significance of physical manifestations.

Difference between Chemistry and Alchemy

In chemistry, if we have the right ingredients and if operations are correctly performed, success will be achieved-independently of the operator.

In Alchemy, even if we have the right ingredients and if operations are properly conducted, success is not necessarily achieved because it depends upon the personal state of the operator. In a very restrictive sense, Alchemy could be viewed as the para physiology of chemistry, for the success of the operation depends upon the inner spiritual state of the operator.

The second difference between the Chemistry and Alchemy is also important. Chemistry doesn't view the bodies it works with as alive. as a matter of fact, the processes are such that chemistry only deals with dead bodies which, of course, can't evolve. Conversely, Alchemy is a biodynamic system which uses the forces of life in its operation. A threefold work is accomplished on bodies: the effects are purification, regeneration and evolution. The most powerful principle are found in the forces of fecundation and reproduction and from these they will be extracted in order to be used. But if this operation seems possible in the vegetable realm, the extraction of the metallic semen or sperm, known only be a few adepts, is considered a Utopian venture by most. The Alchemist or the skilled artist can and must accomplish, through physical material, the manipulation of the divine, spiritual and invisible components which are, in beings and things, the genuine elements of life. Karl von Reichenbach (1788-1896) opined that the existence of a universal power that penetrated all things in the cosmos. The notion was a common one in occult circles in the nineteenth century and was often discussed in terms of aura, astral bodies, animal magnetism, or animal and vegatable electricity. Reichenbach thought that such energy could actually be seen by "sensitive" individuals in the form of light radiation from objects in a darkened room. He called such appearances "Od" after the all piercing power of the germanics God Odin. Spagyric is a unique and harmonious blend of herbal medicine, homeopathy, aromathatheraphy and mineral therapy for holistic healing, a therapeutic treatment that heals body, soul, and the spirit at the same time. Unlike other natural therapies, it focuses on the real cause of the ailment, making it possible to understand why a person became ill and thus leading to a more complete healing. This idea is also the foundation of ancient therapeutic ways of healing, such as traditional Chinese, Tibetan and Ayurvedic medicines. Spagyric presents to modern practitioners a large variety of remedies for all facets of human ailments. In contrast with traditional plant remedies, spagyric is totally non toxic and without any side effects.

Paracelsus (1493-1541) coined the word "spagyric" from two Greek words meaning "separate" and "reunite",alluding to the specific preparation process of a spagyric essence. During this process, the constituents of the plant will be separated, transformed, purified and recombined by methods inspired by Alchemy concepts. the resulting spagyric essence is natural and pure and possess a full spectrum of healing properties for the entire human being. The main difference between a spagyric essence and "classic" herbal tincture is the immaterial healing force developed in the production process of a spagyric remedy. this leads to a higher grade of efficiency. Chemistry is what is called Rasayana in Hindu philosophy, which is physical, but, Alchemy is something very unique, heavenly or spiritual.

13

Pharmaceutical Process

1. **Collection:** It is the gathering of the required drug materials. Exotic drug materials are imported from abroad if there substitutes are not available in the concerned country.
2. **Identification:** By mean of a Botanist, a drug must be examined microscopically as well as chemically too.
3. **Quality Inspection:** Proper physical and analytical procedures must be done to ascertain the quality of drugs, with the aid of suitable instruments and reagents and by chromatography too.
4. **Preserving.** If necessary, drugs and medicinal preparation should be properly preserved in accordance with their properties.
5. **Standardization:** Drugs so prepared are made to conform some standards as per the procedure given by the approved scientific committee.
6. **Combining:** Process of joining two or more things together in a scientific way.
7. **Compounding:** The method of uniting two or more different elements or constituents together so as to form an altogether new product. This new product will have new properties different from those of its constituents. This will produce a "Chemical Compound".
8. **Preparation:** It includes the preparation of Spagyric Essence.
9. **Quality control:** It reveals that whether the drugs and the medicines, so prepared from the ingredients are up to the standard so prescribed in the official Pharmacopoeia. As well as it also includes the use of standard equipments and

laboratory space and environment and preservation of drug and medicine.

10. **Dispensing:** It means preparing and serving the medicinal preparation in accurate way according to the directions of qualified physicians.

14

Laboratory Apparatus

A manufacturing utility of plant alchemy should be spacious enough providing separate departments of:

1. Manufacturing
2. Bonded Laboratory
3. Analytical Laboratory
4. Cloak rooms
5. Finished Products
6. Packing Departments
7. Administration.

In addition to these there should also remain sufficient space required for inter- departmental free movement. The laboratory should be provided with burning gas, electricity and enough quantity of water for washing and cleaning purposes.

List of General Apparatus

a. Coffee filter paper
b. Cotton balls
c. Paraffin
d. Quart Amber bottle
e. Quart Corning Glass pot
f. Faucet Adapter
g. Clamps
h. Stands

i. Coors porcelain crucible
j. Funnels assorted sizes
k. Glass stir rods
l. Graduated Glass Beaker m. Kiln
n. Distillation Train
o. Mortar and pestle
p. Portable electric stove
q. Soxhlet Extractor
r. Mason jars
s. Flasks
t. Test tubes
u. Misc. equipments as per requirement.
v. Microscopes

In a laboratory, evaluation data is generated, measured, calculated or assessed by automatic, mechanical or electronic or computerised equipment. The equipment should be of appropriate design and of adequate capacity to function according to protocols. Examples of such equipments include balances; calorimeters; spectrophotometers; pH meters; refract meter; analytical equipment computerised equipment for direct capture of data. The equipment should be suitably located for operation, inspection, cleaning and maintenance, it is to be assured that the equipments are performing their intended functions. The equipment should undergo validation process for proper functioning.

15

Vehicles Used in Plant Alchemy

The meaning of term "vehicle' is "means of conveyance or transmission". In Alchemy vehicle are the substance, in which medicine are prepared or mixed and provided for -administrations by mean of internal or external application.

Vehicles are an inert substance having no therapeutic value which is used in the preparation of spagyric essence. In Alchemy the vehicles are used in preparation of tincture Aqueous fortes (Spagyric essence of medicinal plants) Vehicles are of dry and fluid consistencies. Plant structures are easily disrupted or rearranged thus destroying the natural synergy. The compounds are easily damaged or destroyed by excessive heat *i.e.* temperatures in excess of 60 Celsius and in some cases even lower. Remember that heat accelerates a reaction. The herb is also sensitive to the type of solvent used to extract its virtues. If the wrong solvent is used it may cause a precipitation reaction whereby the molecules clump and are thrown out of solution; Or worse still the constituents complex, and rearrange themselves into different entities. Consequently the temperatures employed and the type of solvent used are of vital importance if the extract is to remain viable. Complexing is also the consequence of the mixing of two or more plant drugs. Consequently such preparations are of dubious antecedents.

An Ideal Solvent

The following factors should be considered when selecting a solvent for use:

Solvent Power (selectivity)

Only the active, desired constituents should be extracted from the plant material, which means that a high selectivity is required.

Boiling Temperature

The boiling point of the solvent is as low as possible in order to facilitate removal of the solvent from the product.

Reactivity

The solvent should not react chemically with the extract, nor should it readily decompose.

Viscosity

A low viscosity of the solvent leads to low pressure drop and good heat and mass transfer.

Safety

The solvent should be non-flammable and non-corrosive, and should not present a toxic hazard; its disposal should not imperil the environment.

Cost

The solvent should be readily available at low cost.

Vapor Pressure

To prevent loss of solvent by evaporation, a low vapor pressure at operating temperature is required.

Recovery

The solvent has to be separated easily from the extract to produce a solvent-free extract.

The most widely used solvents are Water and Ethanol, followed by Glycerine, organic solvents such as hexane, acetone are also used.

An Ideal Vehicle

1. It must not have any medicinal property of its own.
2. It should be chemically neutral; neither acidic nor alkaline in medicinal effects.

They must not undergo any change or decomposition.

3. The above two specific properties are more applicable to those which are used in potentising medicines.
4. It must be harmless regarding its action on human organisms. The pharmacological message of the original drug is not disturbed in any way.
5. It should be capable of carrying the dynamic powers of drugs into interior human organisms to fight the disease force.
6. It should be edible and palatable.

Liquid Vehicles

In plant alchemy, following liquid vehicles are used:

Aqua Distillata

Specific gravity: 1.000 at 25°C

Boiling point: 100°C

Freezing point: 0°C

Latent heat of fusion at melting point: 79.72 cal / gm

Latent heat of vapourization at boiling point: 539.4 cal / gm

Heat of formation at 25°C: 68.32 Kcal / mole

Critical temperature: 374.2°C

Surface tension at 25°C: 71.97 dynes / cm

Viscosity at 25°C: 8.937 millipoises

Refractive index nD20: 1.333

pH: 5.8 - 7.0

It is a very good solvent, having a physiological inertness, and is one of the most important vehicle in Alchemy. There are three degrees of purity, *e.g.* 'ordinary water', 'purified water' and 'water for injection'. In Alchemy properly purified water may also be used; which should be freshly prepared for use, and be sterile. It must be free from all bacteria and micro-organism.

Alcohol

Chemical Formula : C2H5OH

Molecular Weight : 46.07

Specific gravity: at 25°C: 0.8075 to 0.8104; at 15.6°C: 0.816 (HPUS - Alcohol Fortior contains about 91 Percent by weight or 94 Percent by volume of ethyl alcohol and about 9 Percent by weight or 6 Percent by volume of water. Its specific gravity at 60oF or 15.6°C is 0.820)

Boiling point: 78.37 °C, but volatilizes even at low temperature

Freezing point: -114°C

Refractive index at 20°C: 1.3637 to 1.3639

Readily inflammable, burning with a blue smokeless flame, highly hygroscopic.

Ethanol

Chemical formula: $C2H6O$

Molecular Weight: 46.06844 g/mol

Specific gravity: 0.787 at 25 °C

Freezing point: -114.1 °C

Refractive index: 1.3611-1.3617 at 20 °C

It is a volatile, flammable, colorless principal type of alcohol with a slight characteristic odour.

Glycerin

Chemical Formula: $C3H5(OH)3$

Molecular Weight : 92.094 g/mol

Specific gravity: 1.255 to 1.266 at 20°C

Boiling point: 290°C at latm. with decomposition, but can be distilled intact in vacuum.

Freezing point: about “36 °F / “37.8 °C corresponding to 60–70% glycerin in water.

Refractive index: 1.471 to 1.473 at 20°C

16

Sources of Medicines

Plant Alchemy or Spagyric medicines are prepared from both exotic and indigenous medicinal plants, which grows in their natural habitats. The flowers, leaves, fruits, buds, roots and barks, etc are collected at the time of their maturity to obtain their highest medicinal contents. Nature has perfected the herb, then so must practitioner perfect the medicines derived from them. This is done by timing, right attitude and good intent. The herb must be gathered at the correct time. The plants are examined for contamination, such as other plants, insects or environmental pollution. Selected plants or parts are used in the preparation of spagyric essences.

The Moon and its position in the Zodiac, as observed from Earth, is integral to plant alchemy. As a star, our own Sun is a relatively small body in comparison with many of those giant stars that make up our Zodiacal belt. The output of electronic matter from those stars is in proportion to their magnitude. The evidence of Radio Astronomy is irrefutable, the output of those stars is received and recorded here on earth. All things are the product of their season in the yearly cycle. According to classic philosophy of plant alchemy medicinal plants must be harvested at the correct phase of the moon in relation to the plant part required. When the plant is opened or operated on, each stage should be done at the astrological time allocated for each operation.Without a knowledge of Astrological science and methods, the production of a true spagyric medicine is not possible.

Some of the sources of the Spagyric medicines are given below:

1. **Whole plants (including root):** *Aconitum napellus, Atropa belladonna, Matricaria chamomila, Chelidonium majus, Solanum dulcamara, Euphrasia officinalis, Ledum lalustre, Pulsatilla nigricans, Ruta graveolens.*
2. **Root:** *Armoracia sativa, Cimicifuga racemosa, Hydrastis canadensis, Caphaelis ipecaauanha, Opercuina turpethum.*
3. **Stem:** *Caulophyllum thalictroides, Podophyllum peltatum, Cannabis indica, Sanguinaria canadensis.*
4. **Bulb:** *Allium cepa, Allium sativum, Zingiber officinale*
5. **Leaves:** *Rhus toxicodendron, Artemisia abrotanum.*
6. **Spores:** *Lycopodium clavatum.*
7. **Bark:** *Euonymus europea, Berberis vulgaris, China officinalis, Withenia somnifera.*
8. **Seeds:** *Stramonium, Croton tiglium, Strychnos nux vomica.*
9. **Fruit:** *Syzygium jambo, Semicarpus anacardium.*

The plants are collected soon as they attain their highest contents of active ingredients.

The plants should be free from insecticides, insect contamination or industrial pollution.

The optimum quality and purity of the plants are ensured through Morphological, microscopical and phytochemical examinations.

Collection of Medicinal Plants

The sources of Spagyric medicines is vegetable kingdom. Plants grown under constant supervision of trained personnel or grown in their natural habitat are collected as soon as they attain their highest contents of active ingredients.

These are graded, inspected and processed upon arrival at the laboratory to retain their freshness as well as the active medicinal contents in their native and stabilized form.

1. **Whole plants (including roots):** These are collected in sunny weather when these are in half flowering and half bud stage.

2. **Leaves:** These are collected before the flowering of the plants. In case of biennial herbs the leaves are collected in the spring time of second year, before he flowers develops from the buds.
3. **Flowers:** These are collected in dry weather, when these are partly in bud and partly in the blossom.
4. **Stems:** These are collected when most of the leaves of the plants are fully developed.
5. **Barks:** These are collected in the early spring for resinous herbs, and for the non resinous herbs, in the autumn.
6. **Roots:** These are collected in the spring in case of biennial herbs, when these are in their full vigour. In case of annual herbs, these are collected early in the autumn, before the ripening of the seeds and form perennial herbs these are collected in the second or third year before the woody fibres develop in them.

17

Preparation of Spagyric Essence

The roots of the spagyric or spagyrism can be traced back thousands of years, a founder can not clearly be defined. The word spagyric was used often synonymously to the term "Alchemic". Spagyric or Plant Alchemy is to be received rather a special branch of Alchemy with which in a special manufacturing process the welfare plant is unlocked and/or transformed.

The spagyric method is of separation, purification and reunification (cohobation), it is constituted with the etymology of the Greek word spagiry (spao+ ageiro) which means to separate and reunite.

Spagyric medicines were originally created by fermenting parts of the wild herbs. This process produced concentrated aromatic solutions that were extracted and separated from the bulk plant matter. After fermentation was completed the,

1. Plant material was distilled in a special device.
2. And the remainder dried and burned up
3. The ashes were extracted and purified via distillation, than recombined with the concentrated solution.
4. As a result the finished spagyric essence contained the mineral constituent parts of the plants.

A spagyric essence is clearly colorless to yellowish and smells very intensively aromatically.

The nature of spagyric essences is subtler than that of spagyric tinctures. They are less 'corporeal' more 'dematerialized' and their effects is more penetrating but very subtle. Everything is subtler than with the extracts or even tinctures. Spagyric essences are therefore considered pure medicines.

Spagyric essences have a much longer life span; a virtually unlimited life span.as for their preparation much experience is required in the art of distillation.

Procedure for obtaining Spagyric Essence

All preparation always contains the three philosophical principles.

1. Mercury
2. Sulfur
3. Salt

These principles are extracted (separation), purified (distillation, incineration, calcinations, evaporation) and then reassembled (reunion or cohobation).

The practical works of the plant alchemy lab whether we mean the inner or outer lab, includes three basic process .*i.e.* separation, purification, and cohobation. These three processes are the basis of the evolutionary process of all alchemical works.

In nature, whenever a plant dies, its body is biodegraded and its essential principles (sulfur+mercury+salt) returns to the earth to be used in the life cycle of other plants. the cycle remain in circulation unless an animal eats the plant, in which case the vibration of the plant are transmitted to a higher level by the alchemical power of the living animal realm. This is an internal or naturally happening to this planet.

But if externally or in the alchemical lab, an herb is separated into its essential principle, the oil, the alcohol and the caput-mortem. Each Principle is then purified by using heat (the fire) through distillation, extractions and calcinations. The final step is cohobation which represents a rebirth on a higher level. Thus the plant is taken out of the bio-degradation cycle and is reborn through the raising of its vibration to a level where it can be used for a higher purpose that is medicine in animal realm.

The medicines which are produced through alchemical methods are more efficient than any other vegetable medicine because they contain the three essential principles in a purified and cohobated state.

The word Spagyric meant separate and reunite. The spagyric manufacturing process as it is used, is based on the work of the Swiss physician Paracelsus (1493-1541) and the advancement by the German physician Carl Friedrich Zimpel (1801-1879). Spagyric after Dr. Zimpel is the bridge between classical Homoeopathy and modern Phytotheraphy and is characterised by characteristics.

The preparation of Spagyric essence after Dr. Zimpel is based on three substantial stages, *i.e.* the fermentation, distillation and the Calcination. Thus both ethereal oils become (flavour materials) and plant-own mineral materials and trace elements won. The advantage of these spagyric essence consists therefore of the fact that they contain organic and inorganic materials.

Reunification of Sulfur, Mercury and Salt

Extraction of Sulfur (Volatile Oil)

This is what we may define core alchemical theory. The difficulty in understanding them arises from their meanings in alchemy compared to common use. These names represent principles and do not refer to the actual substances of salt, sulfur and mercury. A primary difficulty in alchemy is that these terms sometimes to mean wildly different things. However, careful examination of the attribution can usually reconcile the disparity.

Mercury is the activating principle of the substance. In Hindu philosophy it corresponds to prana. In plant spagyrics, we note that alcohol can be fermented out of most plant substances. Ethanol is chemically the same whether it is distilled finally out of grapes, potatoes, corn or dandelions. However, the fine distinctions between these alcohols are important in alchemy. Alchemical Mercury is not absolutely identical with ethanol.

On the human level, Mercury corresponds to the part of the human soul that partakes of a Universal Divinity: this is the substance that makes a person alive. Spiritually advanced people concentrate and purify this substance rather than just being content with the share they are given at birth.

Sulfur is the individuality of an entity (plant, animal or human). The Sulfur of an herb is most concentrated in its essential oils. This is its "soul," as it were. In a human being, this would correspond to your unique personality.

Salt is the physical matrix in which the individuality of the substance resides. It is the physical substance of a plant, or the body of a human. When the substance or human is completely dead, only the Salt remains.

Thus, if we extract juice out of grapes, the flavoring and oils would be related to the Sulfur component, the ethanol resulting from fermentation would be the Mercury, and the skins and other parts of the grape that remain behind would be the Salt.

Extraction of Sulfur (Volatile Oil)

1. Steam distillation performed to the crude drug to obtain the volatile oils. Take a 5000ml round bottom flask into a sand bath and poured 3000ml of distilled water into the flask. Take another wide mouth double jointed flask and place a small piece of filter paper inside the flask over the bottom joint. Now add enough grounded herb to the flask so it is half full. Next, hook up the reduction head and the distillation adapter. At last use a 2000ml flask as a receiver at the end of the apparatus.
2. Turn the heat on low after some time, steam will colored up the double-jointed flask as it passed through it. The distillation adapter also will become fogged. At the end of the drip tip there will we see that water droplets are forming. The drops will fall into the receiver. After few milliliters have collected in the receiver, there will be colored oil is collecting on top of the water and when approximately 1500ml of the water has been distilled off, turned off the heat and let the apparatus cool. Then transfer the water and oil in the receiver into the oil separator.
3. Took the double-jointed flask off of the distillation flask. Poured 100 ml of the fresh distilled water into the distillation flask and hook up the entire apparatus. This entire process should be done at least three times to ensure that the majority of the volatile oils come out of the plant body.

Collection of Volatile Oil

4. While the second separation of the sulphur is under way, gather the oils obtained from the first. To do this, simply open the stopcock at the end of the drain tube. Slowly drain off the water, when only a little water is left in the separator, close the stopcock. After each subsequent extraction of the volatile oils from the plant body, take what is in the receiver and place it in the oil separator leaving the oil behind. Reuse this water for all other subsequent separations of oil from the plant body.

Extraction of Mercury

5. Take the essence from the depleted body of the herb and place it into the wide mouthed 5000ml round bottom flask. The water that was left from the separation of the volatile oils is now poured over the herb. Seal up the round bottom flask with a fermentation lock and placed it in an incubator at 27 degree centigrade. In about two weeks, the plant body will have fermented and yielded up its spirit, *i.e.*, Mercury. Distill off the spirit and rectify it seven times. Save the phlegm from the spirit for later use.

Extraction of Salt

6. Take a glass pot and empty the remaining liquid and plant body left in 5000ml flask. Take the pot out door and boil off all the moistures. When the moisture is gone, the herb body will begin to roast, than incinerate it. When the body will obtain an ash grey color, turn off the heat and let the pot cool. Grind and weigh the ash set up the soxhelt extraction and extract the water-soluble salts from the ash. Evaporate the water from the salts in the oven overnight. Grind and weigh the salts, than place them into the kiln to calcine at 600 degree centigrade for one week. At the end of the week, turn the kiln off and let it cool. grind and weigh the salts. repeated the process of extracting, drying, grinding, weighing, claiming, grinding and weighing two more times to get the hygroscopic salt, the third principle (ingredient).

Calcination

7. On completion of the extraction, the residue is pressed and the resulting liquid added to the extract. The pressed residue is then spread out in a fireproof dish and steadily heated from below. Unless one has access to a fume hood, this process is best carried on outdoors because of the volume of smoke and fumes produced. The temperature for the Calcination process should not be allowed to exceed 400 C, let the salts melt and fuse. The Calcination will proceed in stages and pass through different colour changes. The first change being the carbonisation of the marc, which is black. Then through different shades of brown and orange, then finally grey, and then white. When no further changes are observed, then the process of Calcination is complete.

Cohobation

8. Once the hygroscopic salt is obtained, next step is cohobation, mix rectified spirit *i.e.*, Mercury (already preserved) with the Salt then add the volatile oil *i.e.*, sulfur.

Digestion

9. Allow the mixture to digest in an incubator at 30 degree centigrade for a week.

   Be sure to slightly shake the container three to five times a day.

Decantation

10. Decant the essence (spagyric essence) from the undissolved salts. It will be seen that the essence is now colored yellow and smells strongly of the herb been used in the operation.

11. One drop in wine or distilled water will yield the full effects of the plant's medicinal nature. Save the remaining salt.

12. The essence is further used for medicinal preparation which is higher in its quality and non toxic in nature.

Circulation

13. The exaltation, or circulation, is the Spagyric equivalent of the Homoeopathic potentisation or succussion process, whereby the liquid being circulated is raised to a higher level of potency.

Essentially, the liquid to be circulated is gently heated to a temperature not exceeding 35C, inside a closed container, usually a pelican. The vapours from the heated liquid will rise and condense in the head of the flask, and then run back into the main body of the flask thus setting up a rhythmic circulation. The expansion head is critical to the operation. A suitable apparatus may be constructed by using a Separating funnel mounted on the top of an Erlenmeyer flask. The flask is connected to the funnel via a cork or rubber bung. The liquid to be circulated is poured into the flask, and the separating funnel, which will double as the expansion head, is mounted on top. The flask is then gently heated from below. To prevent any damage to the extract, the flask should be suspended in a water bath and the temperature regulated by means of a thermostat. A seven fold circulation is required, *i.e.*, a 7 day process. The apparatus is turned off at night and turned on again during the day. At the end of the seven fold circulation the extract may be considered ready for use.

18

Spagyric Essence by Cohobation Method

Paracelsus provides an old method for a partial extraction in his book "*Book of Archidoxes*"

> "... *herbs and their similar have to be taken first and to be macerated and digested in spirits, during one month. Then distill them in a bain-marie during one month adding plants and separate them : you have a magisterium of the herb you wish to.*"

Cohobation in "Plant Alchemy" is the assembling of the purified elements got by mean of spagyrism. It is not concern to the act of passing again and again a solvent over a substance to open it and to dissolve it as per the definition given by Glaser's.

Thus the process of reassembling the three purified principles (Salt+Sulfur+Mercury) constituted Cohobation or reunification.

According to Jonathan Michael Code of Rudolf Steiner University, Cohobation is followed by 'Exaltation', after 'alchemical marriage' of the three principles, whereby they are re-combined or re-synthesized, which raises the essence to a new energetic level through repeated circulation the liberation is achieved. The processes involved are distillation and cohobation (redistilling with the residues), opined by Johann Valentin Andreae of DePauw University, Indiana, USA. Luigi Vernacchia summerized it as 'alchemical potentization' or 'Cesare Mattei's fixing of plant electricity'.

In alchemy, the meaning of words often has no sense with the meaning usually given to them. The three principles sulphur, mercury and salt have nothing in common with what is generally understood by these words.

All things and all beings possess sulphur, mercury, and a salt: these are principles which concentrate spiritual energies. The sulphur concentrate the soul's energies, the Mercury the spirit energies and the Salt the body energies.

Before cohobating these three principles, have to separate which is always known as the great secret of the plant alchemy.

In vegetable realm, the spirit is contained in the Alcohol and is common to all plants and released by all plants during the fermentation process (death) of the body. The spirit/Mercury is the life force of the cosmos and its vital essence, and represents the major points of interest in Alchemy. The soul of the vegetable world is the essential oil which plants possess to various degree. The soul (Sulfur) is the consciousness of three world (kingdom).The Body (Salt) of the vegetable world is what remaining after the spirit has left. It is also called caput-mortem (dead Head). It is then burnt until it turns into ashes and finally to white salt.

Cohobation is certainly a delicate operation. However, if the Sulfur and the Salt have been purified, the cohobation between then occurs equal weight to equal weight. As for the Mercury, it should only imbibe the others two. Only by carefully watching the process, we can justify that if there is too much or too little mercury.

Various alchemists failed in there experiments for the simple reason because they do not know the theory or do not understand what is happening during experiments. we never get the desired results if we deals the alchemy as applying a textbook. When we don't understand, what we are doing, we kill the subtle principles and we move from alchemy back to chemistry.

There are three levels of the living body, *i.e.* material or molecular level, the information level, and the spiritual level. And Spagyric medicines alone (consisting the three principles) are the perfect medicine in the world to act on the three mentioned levels of the body.

In alchemy after the Cohobation the product undergoes a long Digestion at a constant temperature or a Circulation. According to Von Bernus definition, the aim and the effect of digestion is to obtain the loosening of the textures of substances to allow their opening and dissolution. This phenomenon must be considered as identical to the one that happens in the stomach of an animal.

Cohobation is a uniquely alchemical process: it is not understood by chemistry, in that a chemist would fail to see the point of it. And yet it is through the Cohobation stage that the Alchemist claims that the three Principles somehow get together and form a Quintessence, a substance which is Spiritually more advanced and greater than the sum of its parts. In the present case, that Quintessence would be a perfected Spagyric tincture.

Spagyric remedies undergo six key steps: separation, purification, distillation, incineration, re-unification and circulation.

1. Separation

Chopped plant pieces are added to yeast, sucrose and distilled water to initiate fermentation. This three-week process produces a natural alcohol intrinsic to the particular plant, resulting in a high quality mother tincture solution that contains vital energy specific to that herb.

2. Purification

This product undergoes repeated filtrations to obtain a solution which is completely free of impurities. Similar to producing a fine wine, this process requires time and precision because new particles created by the plant tincture during the various filtering phases must be removed to achieve an absolutely pure liquid solution.

3. Distillation

Next the residue is further added to distilled water, which undergoes steam distillation process.

4. Incineration

In step three, the original plant material used to produce the mother tincture solution is dried, caked and burned at very high temperatures, creating an ash. Which is added to distilled water and filtered to remove all impurities or heavy metals from the ash, the filtered solution is then heated to get the salts or crystals of the plant.

5. Re-unification

Finally, the pure plant crystals — which stimulate metabolic process in the body are combined with the solutions obtained through steps 2 and 3. As the crystals are added to the solutions, a dramatic color change takes place and the specific aroma distinctive to the plant flows from the fluid creating the "miracle" of spagyrics.

All preparations always contain the 3 philosophical principles *i.e.* Mercury, Sulfur and Salt. The principles are extraction, purification and then reassembled.

1. Extraction of the volatile oil (alchemical sulfur).
2. Second distillation "mineralized" mercury (the spirit part).
3. The salt (ash) is added to the distillate.

The first step in the spagyric process is to extract the essence from the plant employed. This essence contains the alchemical Mercury of the plant with its Sulfur adhering to it. The remaining plant matter contains the plant's Salt property.

Apparatus Required

Coffee filter paper

Cotton Balls

Label

Notebook

Empty vessels

Funnels

Sand

Distillation tube

Oil separator

Mortar and pestle

Round bottom flask-5000ml

Round bottom flask-2000ml

Portable Electric stove

Principle

All preparations always contain the 3 philosophical principles *i.e.* Mercury, Sulfur and Salt. The principles are extraction, purification and then reassembled.

Extraction of the Volatile Oil (Alchemical Sulfur)

Procedure

The first step in the spagyric process is to extract the essence from the plant employed. This essence contains the alchemical Mercury of the plant with its Sulfur adhering to it. The remaining plant matter contains the plant's Salt property.

Now we can do the spagyric process by the following steps:

Step 1

The appropriate herb is first ground to a fine consistency, either with a motor or by rubbing it firmly between the hands (here is the process of Maceration).

The ground herb is then placed in a suitable glass vessel, one with a tight lid and covered with the liquid (menstrum), which will extract the essence.

Step 2

We will have to put the herb's essence through a stem distillation. Place a 5000ml round-bottom flask into a sand bath. Next hook up the reduction head and the distillation adapter. Pour 3000ml of distill water into a flask and add enough herbs to the flask so it's half full. Finally, use a 2000ml flask as a receiver at the end of the apparatus. Create a vacuum and distill off most of the liquid. After some time we will see the steam clouding. Our distillation adapter also will become fogged. At the end of the drip tip, we will see water droplet forming. The droplet will fall into the receiver. When approximately 1500ml of the water has been distilled over, turn off the heat. Let the apparatus cool and transfer the water and oil in the receiver into the oil separator.

Step 3

Pour 1000ml of fresh distill water into the distillation flask and hook back the entire process. Repeat the process 10-12 times. The water will now smell mildly of the herb. The essential oils contained in the plants are now in the water. After the last distillation, let the apparatus cool.

Step 4

While our second separation of the volatile oils (alchemical sulfur) is under way, we will gather the oils obtained from the first.

To do this, simply open the stopcock at the end of the drain tube. Slowly drain off the water. When only a little water is left in the separator close the stopcock. After each subsequent extraction of the volatile oils from the plant body, take what is in the receiver and place it in the oil separator. Drain the water out of the separator leaving the oil behind. Reuse this water for all of your subsequent separations of oil from the body.

Step 5

Take the essence, depleted body of the herb and place into the wide mouthed 5000ml round-bottom flask. The water that was left from the separation of the volatile oil is now poured over the herb. The most common menstrum is any form of strong alcohol (about 40 per cent alcohol). The vessel is now sealed and set aside in a worm place about 27 degree C to allow the menstrum to do its work.

After 2-3 weeks, the menstrum will have taken on the greenish hue of the herb, showing that it has achieved the extraction of the essence. Distill off the spirit (alchemical Mercury) as described in the following and rectify it seven times. This is the herb's essence containing its properties of Mercury and Sulfur. Save the phlegm from the spirit for later use.

The remaining herbal matter, containing the salts of the herb, is placed in a flameproof dish for later use.

Step 6

Now it is the time for separation of salts of the plant. Take the remaining herbal matter in a flameproof dish and ignited. Separation of salts follows the following steps:-

Incineration

The incineration of the herbal matter to drive off the carbons and all superfluities to obtain the black ashes wherein is hidden our precious salts. Our sulfur is also driven off with this incineration. As it will burn readily and quickly reduces to black ashes.

Calcination

Solomon Trismosin says "Heat turns all black things white." This is our calcinations to remove the darkness from our matter. These black ashes are than repeatedly heated and ground until they become a light colored powder. This is the process of Calcination.

Manipulation of the Ashes

As our ashes become more and lighter in color, so does the volume diminish as the impurities are continuously driven off back to their source in nature. Grind and weigh the ash.

When we are satisfied with the light colored of our ashes we then dissolve them in distilled water to separate the soluble salts from the insoluble salts.

Leaching out the Soluble Salts

The insoluble salts precipitate to the bottom of our water bottles leaving a milky water ladened with the soluble white salts. We siphon off this salty milky water and preserve it. We dissolve over and over the ashes until all our soluble salts have been extracted leaving behind the "Caput Mortem".

Evaporation

Through the evaporation produced by the heating, we reclaim our soluble salts. They coagulate and emerge from the bottom of our vessel as the waters slowly recede. A very gentle heat and a slow process through hours and days is required so as not to lose some of our salts into the air with the evaporation.

Emerging Salts

At the final stages of the developing of our salts, the very gentle heat of an alcohol burner is enough. The crucible size is always altered for proper size which is important for proper operation.

Nearing the end we must stir continuously and vigorously so as to prevent spitting and splattering. We must remove our salts before they become rock hard so that we may more easily render them into powder form in the mortar.

Second Dissolution

These soluble salts are once again dissolved in hot distilled water to ensure that all the darkness has been removed from our salts. As can be seen to our surprise, more dark ashes have separated and precipitated to the bottom of the bottle. The whole process of the "Evaporation" is again repeated as before.

Whitened Salts

At this point the purity of our salt is ensured and it can be seen by the bright whiteness of the powdered salts. When performed for the first time one cannot help but be amazed by such a purity. A little taste of these salts proves themselves to be very active. An exhilarating and heating action is felt instantly on the tongue.

The Exalted Salts

The ancient alchemists have discovered that matter can be volatilized and exalted. They have found ways to spiritualize matter to make it be fitting as a proper vehicle for the higher forces of nature. "It ascends from earth to heaven and acquires the power of the above...." To us these salts are sacred and ready to be used as a vehicle for manifestation, to perform the bonding to our purified sulfur and mercury.

Step 7

The salt is then recombined with the alchemical mercury and sulfur by placing the salt into the vessel containing the essence and tightly sealing the vessel to prevent the escape of any vapor. The vessel is then set aside in a warm place (at about 27-30 degree C) for about 2 weeks to allow the liquid essence to "digest" the salts of the calcinated ashes. This process is called "digestion". This completes the manufacturing process and the herbal elixir and medication are ready for use. One drop in wine or distilled water will yield the full effects of the plant's medicinal nature. By using this unique method of preparation, spagyric practitioners maintain that the elixir produced is more potent and efficacious than any other form of herbal medicines.

Theodore Krauss postulated cohobation as a form of cold distillation process with fermentation that retained the living, radio-active powers of the plants by accumulating or suspending them in the obtained essence. He recommended to gather the shoots, seeds, branches, leaves, blossoms, fruit, bark, bulbs or roots of the plants one needed in the spring or autumn, when the juices of the plant organism were active, extract their juices by making incisions and soak them in distilled water (maceration) at 35 °C. After that, one had to keep macerating fresh plant material, not in water, but in that solution. The solution gained more and more medicinal substance in the process until full saturation was achieved.

The tincture should then be poured into big glass containers, called recipients, where it remained until it was completely clear; as a result of the fermenting process the impure substances would settle on the ground of the recipient as sludge, while the pure, clear essence contained all the medicinal properties of the plant in a refined, "virtually spiritualised"form, but without the ballast of the plant body and only bound to a small amount of water. (Pathways of Homoeopathic Medicine: Bettina Blessing, Institute for the History of Medicine, Robert Bosch Foundation, Stuttgart, Germany).

As per Hermetic philosophy, Cohobation (elevation) is the rejoining of distillate to it's source for further distillation or co-habitation after marriage of the opposites or the three purified prima materials. Which is achieved through repeated distillations in which the distillate is repeatedly reunified with the residue, and the distillation is carried out a new. Through continual changes in the aggregate conditions of the distillate and through the reunification with the residue in the distillation container, the distillate attains a high level of purity and, at the same time, its effectiveness is dynamised. (Hermetic library article; "Spagyric Elixirs Pt. 3: Further Calcination and Cohobation").

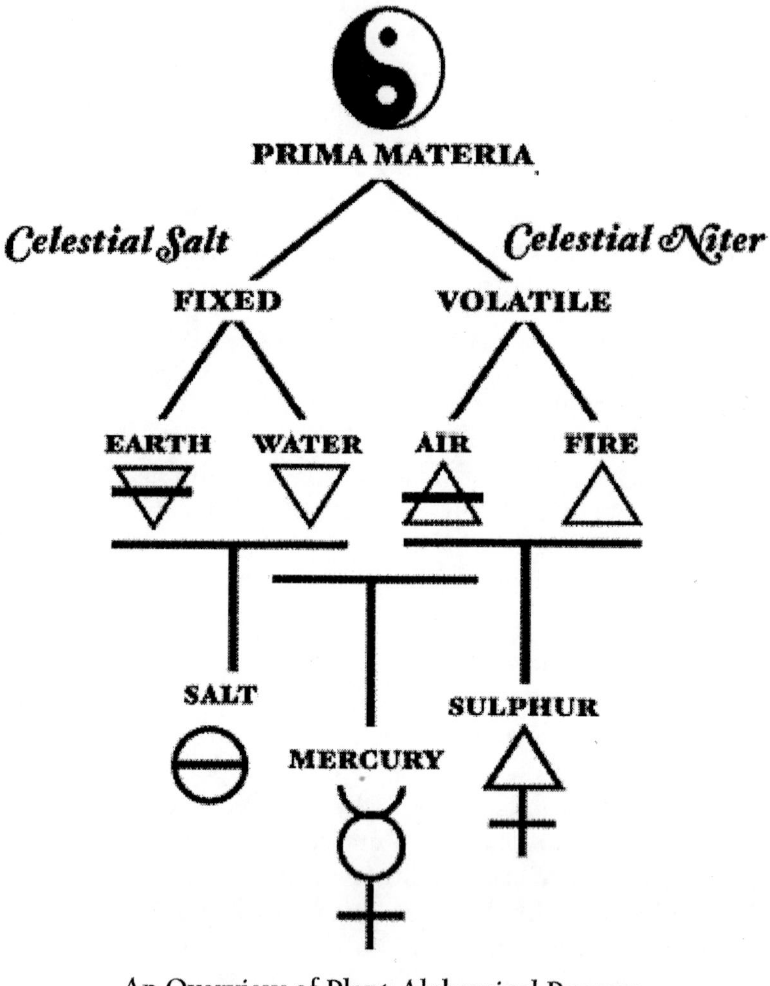

An Overview of Plant Alchemical Process

19

Phytochemical Analysis of Plants

Extraction and Phytochemical Analysis of Plants

Nineteenth century witnessed some real progress in methods of extraction of plant materials for industrial use, *viz.*, in extraction processes which led to the isolation and characterization of many groups of plant metabolites of therapeutic importance, including both single chemical constituents as well as standardized extracts of crude drugs. In manufacturing various classes of medicinal plant preparations, such as decoctions, infusions, fluid extracts, tinctures, semisolid extracts and powdered extracts, popularly known as galenicals, both simple traditional methods and advanced technologies are used, conforming to the official procedures and specifications as laid down in various pharmacopoeias.

Maceration, percolation and infusion are the general techniques used for the extraction of medicinal plants and are mostly applied for galenical preparations. The sole purpose of such basic extraction procedures is to obtain the therapeutically desirable portion and eliminate the inert material by treatment with a selective solvent known as menstrum. These techniques also play a decisive role in the qualitative and quantitative evaluation of the extracts. The standardized extracts thus obtained are further processed for inclusion in other solid and semisolid herbal dosage forms.

The general principles and mechanisms involved in maceration, percolation and infusion for the extraction of the crude drugs are same as to those for the extraction of soluble constituents from solid materials using solvent, which is generally referred to as leaching. The processes of leaching may involve simple physical solution or dissolution. The extraction procedures are affected by various factors, namely the rate of transport of solvent into the mass, the rate of solubilization of the soluble constituents by the solvent, the rate of transport of solution out of the insoluble material. The extraction of crude drugs is mostly favored by increasing the surface area of the material to be extracted and decreasing the radial distances traversed between the solids (crude drug particle). Mass transfer theory states that the maximum surface area is obtained by size reductions which entail reduction of material into individual cells. However, this is not possible or desirable in many cases of vegetable material. It has been demonstrated that even 200 mesh particles contain hundreds of unbroken cells with intact cell wall. Therefore, it is pertinent to carry out extraction with unbroken cells to obtain an extract with a high degree of purity and to allow enough time for the diffusion of solvent through the cell wall for dissolution of the desired solute and for diffusion of the solution (extract) to the surface of the cell wall.

Medicinal Plant Extracts

Extraction, as the term is used pharmaceutically, involves the separation of medicinally active portions of plant or animal tissues from the inactive or inert components by using selective solvents in standard extraction procedures. The products so obtained from plants are relatively impure liquids, semisolids or powders intended only for oral or external use. These include classes of preparations known as decoctions, infusions, fluid extracts, tinctures, semisolid extracts and powdered extracts. Such preparations popularly have been called galenicals, named after Galen, the second century Greek physician. The purposes of standardized extraction procedures for crude drugs are to attain the therapeutically desired portion and to eliminate the inert material by treatment with a selective solvent known as menstruum. The extract thus obtained may be ready for use as a medicinal agent in the form of tinctures and fluid extracts, it may be further processed to be incorporated in any dosage form such as tablets or capsules, or it may be fractionated to isolate individual chemical entities such as ajmalicine, hyoscine and vincristine, which are modem drugs. Thus, standardization of extraction procedures contributes significantly to the final quality of the herbal drug.

Maceration Processes

The general process of maceration on a small scale consists of placing the suitably crushed plant material, or a moderately coarse powder made from it, in a closed vessel and adding the selected solvent called menstruum. The system is allowed to stand for seven days, with occasional shaking. The liquid is then strained off and the solid residue, called marc, is pressed to recover as much occluded solution as possible. The strained and expressed liquid thus obtained is mixed and clarified by filtration. Plant material in fine powder form is never used, as it makes subsequent clarification of the extract difficult. In the case of vegetable drugs, sufficient time is allowed for the menstrum to diffuse through the cell wall to solubilize the constituents within the cells and for the resulting solution to diffuse out. As the system is static, except for occasional shaking, the process of extraction works by molecular diffusion, which is very slow. Occasional shaking assists diffusion and also ensures dispersal of the concentrated solution accumulating around the surface of the particles, thereby bringing fresh menstrum to the particle surface for further extraction. A closed vessel is used to prevent evaporation of the menstrum during the extraction period and thus avoids batch to batch variation. At the end of the maceration process, when equilibrium has been reached, the solution is filtered through a cloth; the marc may be strained through a special press. The concentrations of active constituents in the strained and expressed liquids, sometimes called miscella, are the same and hence they can be combined. The expressed liquid may be cloudy with colloidal and small particles, and sufficient time (perhaps several weeks) is necessary for coagulation and settling. The settled matter is filtered through a filter press or any other suitable equipment.

Percolation

Percolation is a process applied to moisten the drug substances which are in dry powder form or dry crushed out plant residue.

Percolator is a tall cylindrical vessel with a conical bottom and a built-in false bottom with a filter cloth. The percolator is

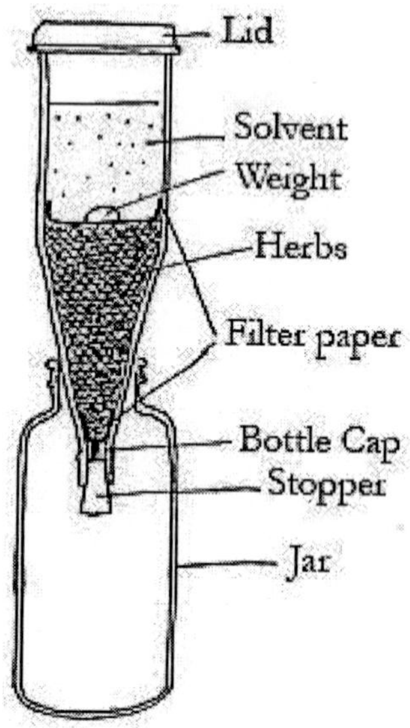

connected to a condenser and a receiver for stripping solvent from the marc. The powdered material is fed into the percolator along with a suitable solvent (ethyl alcohol or another non-polar solvent). The material is left in contact with the solvent until equilibrium of the active principle is achieved. The solvent extract, known as miscella, is taken out from the bottom discharge valve of the percolator. Fresh solvent is added into the percolator and the miscella is drained out after acquiring equilibrium. Overall, the plant material is washed four to five times until it gets exhausted. All washes from the percolator are pooled and concentrated. The solvent in the marc is stripped out by passing steam from the bottom of the percolator. The solvent and steam vapors rise and are condensed in a tubular condenser. The condensate, which is a mixture of alcohol and water, is collected in a receiver and then subjected to fractional distillation to get 95 per cent pure ethyl alcohol which is again used as a fresh solvent.

The maceration period should be kept 24 hours to allow the solvent to diffuse through the drug, solubilize the constituents and leach out the soluble material. In this way, the extraction is more efficient than carrying out percolation without the maceration period. After the maceration, the outlet is opened and the solvent is percolated at a controlled rate with continuous addition of fresh solvent. The volume of percolate collected depends on the nature of the final product. In general, about 75 per cent of the volume of the finished product is collected, the marc is pressed and the expressed liquid is added to the percolate, giving about 80 per cent -90 per cent of the final volume. After assay, the volume is adjusted with calculated quantities of fresh menstrum. If no assay is available, the volume is adjusted after adding the other constituents, if any. In percolation, the expressed liquid is devoid of active constituents as they are already extracted during the percolation period; pressing the marc is only to recover the valuable solvent. This is in contrast with maceration in which the marc is pressed.

Aqueous Alcoholic Extraction by Fermentation

Some medicinal preparations adopt the technique of fermentation for extracting the active principles. The extraction procedure involves soaking the crude drug, in the form of either a powder or a decoction, for a specified period of time, during which it undergoes fermentation and generates alcohol in situ; this facilitates the extraction of the active constituents contained in the plant material. The alcohol thus generated also serves as a preservative. If the fermentation is to be carried out in an earthen vessel, it should not be new: water should first be boiled in the vessel. In large-scale manufacture, wooden vats, porcelain jars or metal vessels are used in place of earthen vessels.

Prahst has mentioned some of the benefits of fermented herbal products which are given below:

1. Fermentation removes most of the undesirable sugars from plant material, makes the product more bio-available and eliminates side effects such as gas and bloating.
2. Fermentation extracts a wider range of active ingredients from the herb than any extraction method since the menstruum undergoes a gradient of rising alcohol levels.
3. Yeast cell walls naturally bind heavy metals and pesticide residues and, therefore, act as a natural cleansing system.
4. Not only does fermentation remove contaminants, it can also lower the toxicity of some of the toxic components in plants.
5. Fermentation actively ruptures the cells of the herb, exposing it openly to the menstruum and bacteria have enzymes that break down cell walls to further assist in the leaching process. Fermentation also creates an active transport system that moves the dissolved constituents from the herbal material to the menstruum.

Soxhlet Apparatus

On the laboratory scale, the Soxhlet apparatus is used. It consists of a flask, a Soxhlet extractor and a reflux condenser. The raw material is usually placed in a thimble made of filter paper and inserted into the wide central tube of the extractor. Alternatively, the drug, after imbibition with menstrum, may be packed in the extractor taking care that the bottom outlet for the extract is not blocked. Solvent is placed in the flask and brought to its boiling point. Its vapours pass through the larger right hand tube into the upper part of the extractor and then to the condenser where they condense and drop back onto the drug. During this period, the soluble constituents are extracted. When the level of the extract reaches the top of the syphon tube, the entire volume of extract syphons over into the flask. The process is continued until the drug is completely extracted. The extract in the flask is then processed. This procedure is thus a series of short macerations.

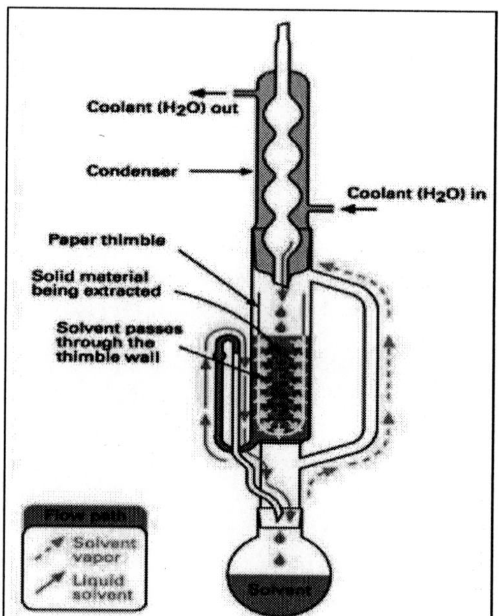

Infusion

The coarsely powdered crude drug (50 g) is moistened, in a suitable vessel with a cover, with 50 ml cold water and is allowed to stand for 15 min. Then, 900 ml boiling water is added, and the vessel is covered tightly and allowed to stand for 30 min. The mixture is strained and enough water is passed to make the infusion measure 1000 ml. Some drugs are supplied (accurately weighed) in muslin bags for preparing specific amounts of infusion and as such are used for infusion preparation. If the activity of the infusion is affected by the heat of the boiling water, cold water should be used. As fresh infusions do not keep well, they should be made extemporaneously and in small quantities at the time of use.

Extraction of Essential Oils

Most essential oils are isolated from the respective plant parts by the process of hydrodistillation or steam distillation. A few essential oils such as those present in the citrus fruit peel can be, and in large part are, obtained by pressing, which yields a product of superior quality. The long action of heat with boiling water affects some thermolabile constituents which may decompose due to hydrolysis, polymerization and resinification. Therefore, the essential oil obtained by distillation does not represent the natural oil as it originally occurred in the plant material. In such plant materials, essential oil is extracted by the process of expression or solvent extraction.

Hydrodistillation

Hydrodistillation is the simplest and oldest process available for obtaining essential oils from plants. Hydrodistillation differs from steam distillation mainly in that the plant material is almost entirely covered with water in the still which is placed on a furnace. An important factor to consider in water distillation is that the water present in the tank must always be enough to last throughout the distillation process, otherwise the plant material may overheat and char. In this method, water is made to boil and the essential oil is carried over to condenser with the steam which is formed. Water-distilled oil is slightly darker in color and has much stronger still notes than oils produced by other methods.

The stills based on this principle are simple in design and are extensively used by small-scale producers of essential oils. Care should be taken during distillation of powdered herbs, as they tend to settle on the bottom of the still and get thermally degraded. Also, for plant material that tends to form mucilage and increase the viscosity of the water, the chances of charring are greater. For plant material that has a tendency to agglomerate or to agglutinate into an impenetrable mass when steam is passed through (like rose petals), water distillation is the preferred method of oil isolation.

Direct Steam Distillation

In direct steam distillation, plant material is distilled with steam generated outside the tank in a steam generator or boiler. As in water and steam distillation, the plant material is supported on a perforated grid above the steam inlet. As already noted, the steam in an FDU is at atmospheric pressure and hence its

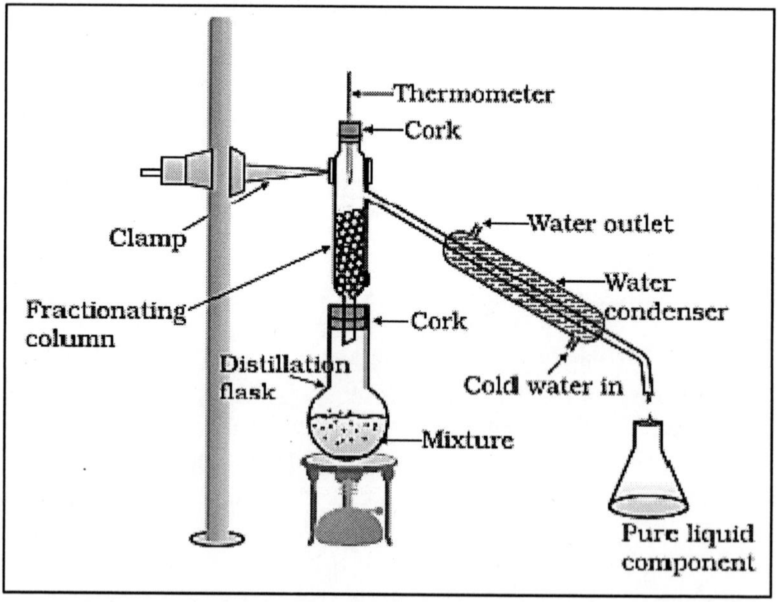

maximum temperature is 100° C. But, steam in a modern pressure boiler operating at, for example, 50 psi pressure will have a temperature correspondingly higher. Moreover, there is no limitation to the steam generation when an external boiler is used as a source of steam. The use of high-pressure steam in modern steam distillation units permits much more rapid and complete distillation of essential oils. Steam distillation is preferred when a lot of area is under cultivation and more than one unit is to be installed. Also, for distillation of high boiling oils and hardy materials such as roots and woods like sandalwood, cedar wood, etc., steam distillation is more efficient. Steam distillation also reduces the time required for the extraction of oils. A charge of Java citronella, which takes up to 5 h in an FDU, is processed within two to 3 h in a steam distillation still. In this method of distillation, steam is generated separately in a steam boiler and is passed through the distillation tank through a steam coil. The plant material is tightly packed above the perforated grid. Steam, containing the oil vapor, is condensed in a tube condenser and is separated in the oil receiver.

Essential oils are a mixture of various aroma chemicals, basically monoterpenes, sesquiterpenes and their oxygenated derivatives, having a boiling point ranging from 150° to 300° C. When the plant material is subjected to heat in the presence of moisture from the steam, these oils are liberated from the plant. For the oil to change from the liquid to the vapor phase, it must receive latent heat that, within the tank, can only come from condensing steam. Consequently, the temperature of the steam within the temperature at which the oil boils in the presence of water on the surface of the plant material, otherwise there would not be a temperature gradient to take the latent heat from the condensing steam to vaporize the oil droplet.

Hand Process

In this process, the freshly harvested fruits are cut transversely into two halves. The pulp is removed with a sharp-edged spoon called rastrello. The peel is then immersed in water for several hours and finally pressed by hand. The worker holds, with the left hand, either one large or two smaller flat sponges on top of a wooden crossbar and, with the right hand, presses the peel against the upper sponge. Thinner peels can be pressed from inside. The emulsion ejected from the oil sacs is soaked by the sponge, which retains solid matter and absorbs colloidal substances. Squeezing the content of the sponge from time to time, oil is finally decanted and drawn off. This process requires much labor and the yield of this method is 50 per cent -70 per cent of the total oil present in the peel. The quality of oil obtained from hand pressing is near to the quality present in fruit peel.

Modern Method

Nowadays, complete mechanization has been achieved and whole fruit processing machines have been developed. These machines either crush whole fruit and then separate the oil from the aqueous phases by distillation or centrifugation, or they express the oil in such a way that it does not come in contact with the juice during the process. The oil extractor developed by Brown International, California, liberates the essential oil from whole citrus fruit. Oil removal is achieved by lightly puncturing the entire surface of the fruit with over three million sharp stainless steel points configured in the form of rotating rolls. An adjustable speed differential between adjacent rolls controls the amount of pressure applied to the fruit. Whole fruits roll across the brown oil extractor, which is made of toothed rollers partially set in a flowing bed of water which propels the fruit across the machine and simultaneously punctures the peel to release the oil from the glands. The fruit proceeds to the extractor and the oil-water mixture goes to centrifugation and to the oil recovery chamber.

Certain high-quality odor-producing flowers such as jasmine, tuberose and gardenia yield small quantities of oil and cannot be distilled by hydrodistillation. Furthermore, the oil components are thermolabile and such flowers, even after plucking, continue to emit small quantities of perfume. The oil from these types of flowers is extracted by cold fat extraction, *i.e.* enfleurage.

Distillation with Cohobation

Cohobation is a technique that can be used for water distillation or for water and steam distillation. It uses the process of returning the distillate water to the still after the oil has been separated from it so that it can be re-boiled. This is basically an improvised methodology of the directly fired type steam and water distillation units for oils which have partial solubility in water.

Although most of the essential oils have finite solubility in water, some oils like those of rose, lavender and geranium have comparatively higher solubility. In such extractions, the loss of oil with the outgoing water of distillation can become alarmingly high. This problem can be solved by returning the condensate water from the separator back to the still; this is known as cohobation. It is evident that this cannot be done with steam distillation as the water level in the still will keep building up due to continuous steam injection. In a further improved version, a packed column is placed on top of the column for providing mass transfer to the oil-water vapors, so as to increase the concentration of the outgoing condensate and to coalesce the oil droplets in the oil separator. The condenser is placed above the column so that the condensate water from the separator can be recycled back to the still by means of gravity. Additional heat, if required, can be provided by a closed steam coil immersed in the tank bottom. The condenser is moved above the distillation still so that condensed water from the separator can flow by means of gravity to the still. By limiting the total quantity of water in this closed cycle operation, it is possible to obtain increased yields of essential oils that are more water soluble. It is relevant to point out here that prolonged recirculation of the distillation water allows the various impurities and plant decomposition products to build up in the system. This may sometimes affect the quality of the oil. One must always keep this in mind when considering a cohobation distillation system for any application.

Thin-Layer Chromatography

Thin-layer chromatography (TLC) is a technique used for identification of medicinal plants and in determining both the chemical composition and biological activity.

It is a simple and efficient method used to identify and quantify secondary metabolites in herbal drugs, its extracts and tinctures, as well as to identify the presence of a secondary metabolite of pharmacological interest in a pharmaceutical formulation. Chromatography procedures are carried out on silica gel, aluminium oxide (alumina) or cellulose plate, these are called stationary phase.

Thin Layer Chromatographic Studies

Glass plates (5 x 20cm) were coated with a uniform layer (0.5 mm) of slurry of silica gel prepared in distilled water using an applicator. After initial drying, the plates were activated in a hot air oven at 110ºC for 30 min. Samples were applied to the adsorbent surface at 2 cm from the edge using a capillary tube and developed in glass chambers (6 x 25 cm) previously saturated with the vapors of the respective solvent system Acetone and Chloroform(7:1) : Acetone and Chloroform (7:3). The plate was removed when the solvent travelled four fifth of the length of the adsorbent on the plate. Visualization was done initially with iodine vapors and observed for any coloration developed and sprayed with suitable chromatographic reagent. Again the plates were activated at 100 degree C for 10 min and observed for any color development, finally visualized under UV light (366 - 254 nm). Three replicates of each sample were examined and mean Rl values were taken.

Column Chromatography:

Retention Factor (Rf) = Distance travelled by the solute from the origin/ Distance travelled by the solvent front from the origin 10 -20g of 60-120 mesh size silica gel was first dissolved in chloroform, then stirred to mix the combination thoroughly to remove the air bubble and then slowly transferred into the glass column, the silica particle settles slowly in the column as stationary phase. The slurry of activated silica was made in and charged in the column in small portions with gentle taping after each addition, in order to ensure packing. A small quantity of solvent was allowed to remain at the top of the column in order to avoid the drying of the column. Tapping is necessary to avoid the air bubble formation in the column during packing which otherwise may interfere in the separation. The packed column was kept undisturbed overnight. Once the column was packed with chloroform solvent mixture was prepared *i.e.*, toluene : chloroform, chloroform: methanol in the ratio 5 : 2, 5 : 1 as mobile phase, mobile was passed through the column for some time and collected at the bottom. 2g of sample to be separated was taken and dissolved in chloroform (may be 1ml of chloroform), the flow rate was set to 10ml/ min. Sample was loaded to the column and eluted with mobile phase. The fraction of 10ml in each tube were collected in a test tube, about

100ml of toluene: chloroform: methanol (30:30:30) was eluted. The column was finally washed with methanol. The fraction was dried and dissolved in known amount of chloroform, TLC was done to find the number of compounds separated.

All the fractions collected through column chromatography was evaporated using rotary evaporator and subjected for TLC. The compound solvency was checked in various solvents like acetone, hexane, benzene, chloroform and methanol. Compound soluble in methanol spotted on an activated TLC plates and separated with a solvent combination of toluene : chloroform: methanol (9 :0.5: 0.5). The TLC plate was kept in iodine chamber for color developing. Eluent 113 th to 129 th have found to be similar in TLC, therefore these were pooled and categorized as fraction FT1, and further subjected for spectral analysis like HPLC, LCMS/MS, FT-IR and NMR.

HPLC

Isolated compound was dissolved uniformly in 100 per cent methanol and 10 µl of sample taken and made upto 1ml in HPLC grade methanol and injected in the HPLC system.

Chromatographic Conditions

Column : Reverse phase C18 (4.6 x 250 mm) 5 µm.

Mobile phase: methanol : water : : 90 :10 v/v.

Rate of flow: 0.2 ml/min

Sample dissolved in methanol

Injected volume : 5 µL

UV -vis wave number 254nm

LCMS/MS

Isolated compound was dissolved in the 100 per cent DMSO, 5µ L of sample is dissolved in 0.5ml methanol and injected in the LCMS/MS system and scanned from 100-1000m/z.

NMR

NMR spectra were recorded on Varian 400 MHz instrument in CDCl and DMSO solutions. Chemical shifts are reported with respect to tetramethylsilane (TMS, delta=0.00 as internal standard (for 1 H NMR) and central line (77.0 ppm) of CDCl 3 (for NMR) expressed in parts per million (delta) downfield from Me 43 Si. Spin multiplicities are given as s (singlet), t (triplet), and m (multiplet) as well as b (board). Coupling constants (J) are given in hertz.

FTIR

Infrared spectra were recorded on a FTIR. From the preliminary phytochemical analysis it is evident that only chloroform fraction contains carbohydrates, glycosides and phytosterols which forms the main constituent in the callus. For further characterization of compounds, chloroform fraction are to be considered.

HPLC and Mass Spectrometric Analysis 2

HPLC stands for high performance liquid chromatography. It is a liquid chromatography which involves the separation of the ingredients on the basis of their polarity. It is used to analyze, identify, purify and quantify the plant materials.

The analysis of the FT 1 was done in High Performance Liquid Chromatographic system (HPLC) equipped with LC8A pump, SPD-M 10 A vp photo array detector in combination with class LC 10 A software Shimadzu, Japan. The chromatographic conditions for the analysis were as follows: mobile phase; Methanol: Water 90:10 v/v, column: ODS (octadecyl silane) Zorbax SB C18 (4.6x250mm) 5 um Detector: SPD-M 10 A vp photo array detector, wave length: 254nm, flow rate: 0.2 ml/min, injection volume: 5 u l. HPLC injections for each of the samples were done at least in duplicate.

The major peak was obtained at the retention time 3 min. The HPLC analysis of FT 1 fraction shows that the peak eluted at 3 min is predominate showing the absorbance at maximum at 210 nm. The same fraction was then passed to the MS to check the molecular weight of the compound.

TLC for Chloroform Fraction FT 1

TLC is used for separation of mixture and identification of constituents using different solvents. Higher the retention speed or low the retention time on TLC plates, better the solvent would be vice versa.

A number of solvents and solvent mixtures were tried. Toluene : Chloroform (9:1); Toluene : Chloroform (3:7); Chloroform : Methanol (9:1) and finally Toluene :Chloroform : Methanol (9:0.5:0.5), v/v/v was found to be the best solvent for separation.

Mass Spectrometry

The mass analysis of FT 1 was studied in LCMS -2010A Shimadzu system equipped with mass hunter software. The sample was run in ESI position scan mode and monitored using single ion monitoring mode. In the presence of halogens the values will show M and M + 2 in positive; M and M -2 in negative. FT 1 fraction gave major peak with a (M + H+) mass of 400.

Plant steroids are collectively known as phytosterols. They are mainly restricted to the plant membranes and may function as cholesterol does in animal membranes. Goodwin and Mercer postulated that evidences for this have been found in some plants where progesterone and deoxycorticosterone were detected. It also showed the analgesic properties and central nervous system activities.

HPLC stands for high performance liquid chromatography. It is a liquid chromatography which involves the separation of the ingredients on the basis of their polarity. It is used to analyze, identify, purify and quantify the plant materials.

A Few Common Laboratory Exercises

Preparation of Extracts

1. Leaf Extraction

a) Aqueous Extract

25 grams of fresh leaf material was macerated with 50 ml of distilled water in a warring blender for 10-15 min. The macerate was first filtered through double layer muslin cloth then centrifuged at 3500 rpm for 30 min. The supernatant was filtered through filter paper and sterilized at 120 C for 15 minutes. The extracts were preserved aseptically at 5 c in airtight bottle until further use.

b) Soxhlet Extraction

Thoroughly washed leaves were dried in shade and then powdered with the help of warring blender. 25 grams of shade dried powder was filled in the thimble and extracted with 100 ml of each of petroleum ether, chloroform, methanol and ethanol successively up to 48 h using soxhlet apparatus. Each of the solvent extracts was concentrated separately using rotary flash evaporator and preserved aseptically at 5 C in airtight bottle until further use.

2. Determination of Ash Values

The ash remaining following incineration of plant materials is by three different methods which measure total ash, acid insoluble ash and water soluble ash.

i) Determination of Total Ash

The total ash method is meant to measure the total amount of material remaining after incineration. This includes both "Physiological ash" which is derived from the plant tissues itself, and "non-physiological ash", a residue of the extraneous materials (sand, soil etc.) adhering to the plant material. 4 grams of the ground air-dried plant material was accurately weighed, in a previously incinerated and tarred silica crucible. The powdered drug was evenly spread as a thin layer at the bottom of the crucible and incinerated by gradually increasing the temperature until it is white indicating absence of carbon. The crucible was cooled in a desiccator and weighed. To get the constant weight the above procedure was repeated. The percentage of total ash was calculated with reference to the air dried drug.

ii) Determination of Acid Insoluble Ash

The ash obtained as described above was boiled with 25 ml of 2N hydrochloric acid for 5-6 minutes and filtered after cooling. The insoluble ash collected on the filter paper was washed with hot water. The insoluble matter was incinerated in a tarred silica crucible which was incinerated and weighed. The procedure was repeated to obtain constant weight. The percentage of acid insoluble ash was determined with reference to the air-dried drug.

iii) Determination of Water Soluble Ash

25 ml of water was added to the total ash obtained and boiled for 5 minutes. The insoluble matter was collected on an ashless filter paper, washed with hot water and incinerated in a crucible

for 15 minutes a temperature not exceeding 450 degree C, weight of the residue was subtracted from the weight of the total ash. Content of water soluble ash was calculated with reference to the air dried drug.

3. Fluorescence Analysis

Fluorescence character of powder plant and callus were studied both in visible light and ultraviolet light (254 nm - shortwave and 365 nm - long wave) by treating the powder material with methanol, methanolic sodium hydroxide, ethanol, ethanolic sodium hydroxide and dilute hydrochloric acid. The organic molecules absorb light usually over a specific range of wavelength, and many of them re-emit such radiations. Such a phenomenon of re-emission of absorbed light that occurs only when the substance is receiving the exciting rays known as "Fluorescence". The fluorescence property of the drug powders was studied under both visible light and ultra violet light.

4. Detection of Chemical Constituents

The extracts of plant material were subjected to quantitative chemical tests for the detection of various plant constituents.

i) Tests for Alkaloids

A small portion of the solvent free extracts was stirred separately with a few drops of dilute hydrochloric acid and filtered. The filtrates were subjected to the following tests to determine the presence/absence of alkaloids.

a) Mayer's test (Potassium mercuric iodide)

The filtrates were treated with Mayer's reagent and observed. The formation of a cream color precipitate indicated the presence of alkaloids.

b) Dragendroff 's test (Potassium bismuth iodide)

The filtrates were treated with Dragendroff 's reagent and observed. The formation of a reddish brown precipitate indicated the presence of alkaloids.

c) Wagner's test (Iodine in Potassium Iodide)

The filtrates were treated with Wagner's reagent and observed. The formation of a yellow color precipitate indicated the presence of alkaloids.

d) Hager's test (Saturated Picric acid Solution)

The filtrates were treated with Hager's reagent and observed. The formation of a yellow color indicated the presence of alkaloids.

ii) Tests for Carbohydrates and Glycosides

Small quantity of extracts were dissolved in 5 ml of distilled water and filtered separately. The filtrates were used for various carbohydrates tests.

a) Molisch's test

The filtrates were treated with solution of alpha napthol, to this and a few drops of sulphuric acid were added through the sides of the test tube. Formation of violet rings indicates presence of Carbohydrates.

b) Fehling's test

The filtrates were treated with few drops of dilute hydrochloric acid and heatedon a water bath for 30 minutes. After hydrolysis the solutions were neutralized with sodium hydroxide, equal quantities of Fehling's A and Fehling s B solutions were added and heated on a water bath for few minutes, formation of red orange precipitate indicates the presence of reducing sugars.

c) Benedict's test

The filtrates were treated with 5 ml of Benedict's reagent and heated on water bath for few minutes. Formation of red orange precipitate indicates the presence of reducing sugars.

d) Legal's test

The hydrolysate was treated with sodium nitroprusside in pyridine and methanolic alkali. Formation of blood red color indicates the presence of cardiac glycosides.

e) Modifid Borntranger's test

The hydrolysates were treated with ferric chloride test solution, immersed in a boiling water bath for 5 minutes and allowed to cool. The cooled mixtures were shaken with an equal volume of benzene. The benzene layer was separated and shaken with about half of its volume of liquid ammonia. The formation of a rose pink to cherry red color in the ammoniac layer tested positive for the presence of anthranol glycosides.

iii) Test for Phytosterols

The petroleum ether, acetone and alcoholic extracts were refluxed separately with solution of alcoholic potassium hydroxide till complete saponification took place. The saponification mixture was diluted with distilled water and extracted with solvent ether. The ethereal extracts were evaporated and residue was subjected to Libermann– Burchards tests.

a) Libermann-Burchard's test

The hydrolysates were treated with a few drops of acetic anhydride, boiled and cooled. A few drops of sulphuric acid were added through the sides of the test tube. Formation of a brown ring at the junction of 2 liquids and green color in the upper layer indicates presence of steroids and triterpenoids).

iv) Test for Oils and Fats

a) Spot test

A small quantity of petroleum ether and benzene extracts were pressed separately between 2 filter papers. Oils stain on the filter paper indicate the presence of fixed oil.

b) Saponification test

A few drops of 0.5 N alcoholic potassium hydroxide were added to a small quantity of petroleum ether or benzene extracts along with a drop of phenolphthalene. The mixture was heated on a water bath for 1 to 2 hours. Formation of soap or partial neutralization of alkali indicates the presence of fixed Oils and Fats.

v) Test for Saponins

a) Foam test

About 1 ml of alcoholic and aqueous extracts were diluted separately with distilled water to 20 ml and shaken in a graduated cylinder for 15 minutes. A centimeter layer of foam indicates presence of saponins.

b) Haemolysis test

The plant extract was diluted with phosphate buffer pH – 7.4. To this 1 ml of 2 per cent blood was added. The test tubes were inverted gently to mix avoiding the formation of foam.

The test tubes were shaken after 30 minutes interval and then allowed to stand at room temperature for 6 hours. Total haemolysis is indicated by a clear, red solution without deposit of erythrocytes.

vi) Test for Phenolic Compounds and Tannins

a) Ferric chloride test

To the test solutions, a few drops of neutral ferric chloride solution was added. The formation of a bluish black coloration indicated the presence of phenolic compounds.

b) Gelatin test

To the test solution, 1 per cent solution of gelatin containing sodium chloride solution was added presence of tannins was indicated by the formation of a white precipitate.

c) Vanillin hydrochloride acid reagent

The test solutions were added with vanillin hydrochloric acid reagent and the formation of a pinkish red color was observed for the presence of Tannins.

vii) Test for Proteins and Amino Acids

a) Biuret's test

To 3 ml of the hot aqueous extract of the plant material 5-8 drops of 10 per cent W/V sodium hydroxide solution was added followed by 1 or 2 drops of 3 per cent W/V copper Sulphate solution. Red or Violet color formation indicates the presence of proteins.

b) Millon's test

A small quantity of the extract of the plant material was dissolved in 1 to 2 ml of distilled water and 5- 6 drops of Millon's reagent was added. The formation of white precipitate turning red when heated indicates the presence of proteins.

c) Ninhydrin test

3 ml of the extract and 3 drops of 5 per cent nynhydrin solution were heated in boiling water bath for 10 minutes and observed for the formation of purplish or blue color.

viii) Test for Gums and Mucilage

a) Alcoholic precipitation test

100 ml of aqueous extract of the crude drugs was slowly added to 25 ml of absolute alcohol with constant stirring and filtered precipitate obtained was dried in air and observed for the presence of gums and mucilage.

ix) Test for Volatile Oil

About 50 g of powdered material was taken in a volatile oil estimation apparatus and subjected to hydro distillation for the detection of volatile oil. The distillate was collected in the graduate tube of the assembly in which the aqueous portion gets automatically separated from the volatile oil and returned to the distillation flask.

x) Test for Flavonoids

a) Shinoda test

To the test solutions, a few fragments of magnesium metal were added along with concentrated hydrochloric acid. On heating the formation of magenta color indicates the presence of flavonoids.

b) Lead acetate test

The extracts were treated with lead acetate solution (10 per cent W/V), yellow precipitate indicates the presence of flavonoid.

c) Ferric chloride test

The extracts were treated with neutral ferric chloride solution, formation of blackish green color indicates the presence of flavonoid.

20

Different Spagyric Methods

Fundamentals of Spagyric is the transformation of matter. The image of alchemists making gold from lead until today characterizes the ideas of this ancient science. The Spagyric as a branch of medical alchemy deals with natural materials such as plants, minerals and metals, high-level remedies to make. By certainly pharmacological techniques, such as fermentation, distillation and ashing, the starting material in a specially converted healing drugs.

The manufacturers spagyrischer medicines rely usually on the traditional writings of the Alchemists and Spagyrists of the Middle Ages and the beginning of modern times. Often, the various systems on prominent personalities of the 19th researchers and early 20th Century are applied in most laboratories. Carl-Friedrich Zimpel (1801-1879), Cesare Mattei (1809-1896), Theodor Krauss (1864-1924) and Alexander von Bernus (1880-1965) were the most important among them.

Spagyrist and philosopher Heilpraktikers Ulrich Juergen Heinz (born 1941) prepared spagyrics of patients blood and used it both as a diagnostic therapeutic ways.

Standardization of Production Rules

In the modern era, some of the spagyrics manufacturing methods have been included into Homeopathic Pharmacopoeia (HAB) and standard procedures have been recorded. Other Spagyric methods are company specific.

The Spagyric methods included in Homeopathic Pharmacopoeias relate to the production of spagyric medicines from plant materials.

Spagyrics after Zimpel

This procedure refers to Carl-Friedrich Zimpel, which he demonstrated in 19th century. The production method of Zimpel-Spagyrics is basically Homeopathic Pharmacopoeia of Germany oriented, however, more techniques have been described by Rudolf Johann Glauber in his "Pharmacopoea spagyrica".

In the Homeopathic Pharmacopoeia of Germany the rules 25 and 26 addressed to the manufacturing of Spagyrics by the Zimpel method, it is also listed in the Homeopathic Pharmacopoeia of the United States.

Fresh or dried plants are crushed and with the addition of water and yeast for fermentation (temperature: 20 to 25° C). When completed, the menstrum is subjected for steam distillation. The distillation residue is dried at a temperature of 400° C. The ashes are added to the distillate followed by a filtration.

The finished medicines, the official name spagyrische mother tincture "after Zimpel" (spag. Zimpel). Traditionally the Spagyric here speaks of "spagyric essence". This can also exponentially after homeopathic scheme, but most undiluted reached on the application. Tinctures from dried plant materials correspond to the 1st Decimal potency (D 1).

Zimpel-Spagyrics are clear liquids highly aromatic, sometimes having peculiar smell. Pharmacologically, it is steam distilled spirits, in which the water-soluble salts from the plant ashes are contained. Toxic substances, such as alkaloids, Glycosides, etc. in the preparations are usually excluded, so even with a poisonous plant question of toxicity does not arise.

Spagyrics after Krauss

This method was developed by Theodore Krauss together with the pharmacist Johannes Sonntag (1863-1945). It refers to the System of "Electrohomeopathy", founded by the Italian Cesare Mattei in the 19th Century. The preparations are still carried out at the Ettlingen based premises of ISO Arzneimittel GmbH(now a subsidiary of Dr. Willmar Schwabe GmbH and Co. KG, Karlsruhe).

In the Homeopathic Pharmacopoeia of Germany the rules 27-30 addressed the manufacturing of Spagyrics by the Krauss method, it is also listed in the Homeopathic Pharmacopoeia of the United States.

Fresh or dried plants are crushed and water, yeast and sugar are added for the fermentation (temperature: 35° C). When completed, it follows an alcoholic extract of the residue through percolation. The menstrum and alcoholic extract is separated to obtain the Spagyrics after Krauss (spag. Krauss).

Spagyrics after Heinz

Ulrich Juergen Heinz developed in the eighties his own spagyrics system, which is still in development and is currently in its latest form "cluster medicine." Heinz processes is listed in German Homeopathic Pharmacopoeia (rule 31).

Fresh plants or plant parts are crushed and water and yeast are added for fermentation (temperature: 18° C). When completed, the menstrum is subjected to steam distillation under a pressure of 3.2 bar. The distillation residue is dried at about 850° C. The mixture of ash and distillate is distilled at atmospheric pressure. Finally filtered and the extract is used as mother tincture.

Spagyrics after Beyersdorff

The procedure is developed by Dr. rer. Nat. Peter Beyersdorff, the founder of pharmaceutical firm Pekana, known for it's homeopathic complex medicines. Homeopathic Pharmacopoeia of Germany govern the manufacturing process under rule 47a and 47 b, also registered under revision of Homeopathic Pharmacopoeia of the United States(HPUS).

Fresh or dried plants are crushed and water, yeast and sugar are added for fermentation (temperature: 20-25° C). When completed, the menstrum is filtered. The residue is dried at a temperature of 900° C. Finally, the ash is added to the extract previously filtered. The final product is called Spagyric mother tincture after Pekana (spag. Peka).

Spagyrics after Strathmeyer

Chemist Walter Strathmeyer (1899-1969)'s process eliminates both the distillation and the calcination processes, and therefore marked as deviated form of spagyrics. Developed by chemist Walter Strathmeyer, Strathmeyer spagyrics is based on the cultivation of yeast fungi. To manufacture its products, he founded the Strath lab, which still produces spagyrics. Homeopathic Pharmacopoeia of Germany regulates Strathmeyer Spagyrics under rule 50 a, b, c.

Dried plants are crushed, and water, special Strath- herbal yeast and sugar are added for the fermentation (temperature: 24-29° C), when completed, menstrum and the liquid Strath-yeast extract are separated by pressing and added ascorbic acid. The final product is labelled as spagyric mother tincture after Strathmeyer (spag. Strathmeyer). Preparations are diluted as per homeopathic potentisation. It is entirely complex preparation.

Spagyrics after Conrad Johann Glückselig

Unless otherwise prescribed, 1 part of starting material is dissolved or dispersed liquid excipient in 99 parts. As excipients Purified water, acids and in "excipients and auxiliaries" section (H 5.3) are used listed ethanol-water mixtures. The solution or mixture is optionally pre-treated and then distilled once to several times, being united after each distillation with the exception of the last with the distillate to the residue. Distillation is considered completed when 100 parts existing in the distillation vessel at the start of the respective distillation solution or mixture 80 or 90 parts of distillate are obtained. The number of distillation and the quantity of distillate is required respectively. The Spagyric of Glückselig gives importance on the steps of fermentation and ashing. Spagyric of Glückselig is governed under rule 54 a, b of German Homeopathic Pharmacopoeia.

Spagyrics after Bernus

Spagyrics after Alexander von Bernus (1880-1965) trace back to the original sources of Parcelsus. Water extractions of various plant arts are fermented at 37° C, without the addition of yeast or sugar. A tincture is obtained through repeated steam distillations of the plant residue, which is also calcinated at high temperatures to obtain ash. Afterward, new plants and products obtained from the extraction (ash, essential oils) are added to the tincture and the "circulations" are resumed. Cosmic influences, such as the position of the sun, moon and planets, as well as rhythmical processes are likewise taken into consideration. These complex remedies are unique in that they also include metallic and mineral elements. The addition of metallic and mineral elements to spagyric remedies is based upon the observations made by earlier spagyric therapists who, through their examination of the laws of correspondence in nature, were able to draw connections between the functions of certain metals and the regulation mechanisms of specific organ systems. Alexander von Bernus, founded Soluna Laboratory, which is still producing Spagyrics after Bernus. A special feature of the Spagyrik after Bernus is spagyrische processing of minerals and metals. The system of the drug after Spagyrik by Bernus complex consists of 28 complexes, of which 23 are for internal use, three ointment preparations, and two blends of essential oils, both internally and externally that can be used. Alexander von Bernus, founded Soluna Laboratory, which is still producing Spagyrics after Bernus. Spagyrics after Bernus is covered under Rule 56 a, b, c, d, e, f, g, h, i, j in GHP as spag. von Bernus.

Non-standardized Spagyric Methods

Besides the above methods governed by Homeopathic Pharmacopoeia of Germany and America, numerous spagyric manufacturing processes are prevailing, which are company specific and hence very specific remedies are produced. The best known are:

Spagyrics after Solitaire

This method has been developed by Achim Stockhardt founder of Solitaire lab, Kirchzell, Germany, it uses the traditional methods of fermentation, distillation and calcination, and also takes into account cosmic cyclical conditions. In addition to spagyric tinctures, spagyric essences, which are cynically handled for an additional 1-1.5 years, are made. Which belong to the true realm of alchemy.

Spagyrics after IFAS

Friedrich Tölle and Wilfried Just founded the Institute for Applied Spagyrik (IFAS) which offers a separate spagyric system. Goal of the institute was originally to revive the Cesare Mattei method. Given this, IFAS developed a unique system in line with Mattei Spagyrics. The IFAS basically use a combined process, the elements of Spagyrics after Zimpel and Spagyrics after Lemasor.

Spagyrics after Lemasor

This process is based on the technique of Thomas Bönschen, who founded the pharmaceutical company "Lemasor" for it's own line of productions. Lemasor Spagyrics are prepared from vegetable source through an alcoholic aqueous extraction process in the full sun and moon light. Simultaneously, from the aqueous herbal menstrum the same plant essential oil is extracted. aqueous-alcoholic liquid is filtered, and dried residue is burned to ash. Lastly, essential oils and ash attached to the aqueous-alcoholic liquid. Spagyrics after Lemasor offers complex medicines.

Spagyrics after Solaris

Karl Spagyrikers Richert has created the Solaris laboratory to produce the lines of preparations after Karl Spagyrikers Richert. For the production of Spagyrics traditional methods such as fermentation, distillation and extraction are obsvered. Besides plants, metals and minerals are also processed. The system of Spagyrics after Solaris consists of twelve complex products. It is based on the two polar-based elixirs therapeutically for the treatment of "negative" and "positive" disease states similar to Mattei.

Spagyrics after Mattei

The spagyric process involves turning a plant material into a tincture, through maceration and pressing, which is fermented for about a month. The tincture is then purified through a series of filtration and distillation (the extract is distilled twice in a glass distiller). The leftover plant material is heated to an ash and filtered with water until crystallization occurs. This indicates that the maximum amount of mineral has been extracted from the plant material. The minerals are then reunited with the finished liquid essence. These ingredients are then converted into low-potency medications, in pills, liquids or simple. The dynamization is carried out by violent shaking (by impact) of the diluted product, to be carried out for at least 100 times in the vertical direction, with net movements, fast and short distance (about 20 centimeters). Mattei Spagyrics is uniquely designed to stabilize and rejuvenate the entire emotional matrix of the patients.

Spagyrics after Junius

Prof. Manfred Junius was born in 1929 in Germany. He was a Professor of Biology at the University of Calcutta. In later years, he opened a spagyric laboratory in Adeleide, Australia. He wrote a modern handbook for plant alchemy, an important contribution to Modern Spagyrics.

Junius prescribed basically a typical alcoholic maceration, the distinctive difference is in the maceration time. Junius prescribed maceration for at least 8 weeks. Thus, the tincture becomes very color intensive and cohesive in the taste. After that, the liquid is poured off, filtered and sealed in a dark glass vessel.

The remaining plant residue is dried, combusted and cleaned in the fire. From the clean ash the mineral salts are drawn and added to the tincture. After the addition of the salts the tincture becomes durable for years without losing quality, whereas, conventional tinctures lose their quality continuously after one year.

Spagyrics as per Indian Alchemy

Cold Fermentation of plant material has been used for the preparation of alchemical medicine. Mud pots are used for the fermentation process: (A) its outer surface is coated with calcium hydroxide, prepared out of kankar lime (CaO); (B) pots placed in the fumes of sambarani (styrex benzoin); (C) precautions are taken to protect from rainwater and other atmospheric contaminants. The plant material is transferred to the prepared pot with boiled cooled molasses water (1:7), and stirred well for 30 minutes with natural yeast. Then the mouth of the pot is closed with a clean cloth to avoid contamination. The upper edge and mouth of the pots are swiped with a cloth (3 cm in width) dipped in castor oil to protect the pot from insects. The pot then kept in sunlight for 168 hours. Then, the pot is kept in a safe place in shade and covered with a lid to protect it from rainwater and dust. After 30 days it is opened, and subjected to steam distillation.

After distillation the liquid and the residue are collected separately. The residue is dried in sunlight and subjected to calcination (parpam, centuram) that was done in mud pots (putankal). These pots were sealed with several layers of cloth strips impregnated of clay, and put to dry. The putankals are filled with dried residue and closed with several layers with cloth strips impregnated of clay. The putankals are dried, then placed in a pit which is filled with dry cow dungs. The cow dungs are lit.

Two days later, the putankal are removed from the pit, opened and the whitened ashes are collected. If necessary, it is grinded until it becomes a very fine powder.

This powder is finally added to the distilled liquid and subjected to circulation, the product is then stored for achieving maturity for 90 days, the final product is then filtered and preserved for medicinal uses.

References:

1. Hans-Josef Fritschi: "Spagyric, Lehr- und Arbeitsbuch", Gustav Fischer Verlag, Ulm 1997.
2. Helmut Gebelein: "Alchemie, Die Magie des Stofflichen", Diedrichs Verlag, Munich 1996.
3. Alexander Roob: "Alchemie und Mystik", Bendikt Taschen Verlag, Colonge 1996.
4. Rudolf Hauschka: "Substanzlehre", Klostermann GmbH, Frankfurt 1990.
5. Peter Schleicher: "Grundzüge der Immun-diagnostik und Immuntherapie", Hippokrates Verlag, Stuttgart 1997.
6. Debasish Kundu: Mysticism, Romance & Secrets of Count Cesare Mattei, LBO Publishing, USA, 2017.

21

Quality Control Procedures

Modern laboratory procedures of quality control neither invalidate ancient precepts nor replace classical procedures.

Indeed, had modern advances in scientific knowledge and equipment been available to the Indian Alchemists, they, in their wisdom would certainly have taken advantage of them. It must be emphasized, however, that ultimately the attainment of a high quality standard is only possible if one could rely on the integrity, the involvement, the training, the commitment of all concerned. This is essentially a team activity with the objective to guarantee the purity, reliability and reproductability supplied to the practitioners.

It must be emphasized, however that ultimately that attainment of a high quality standard is only possible if one could rely on the integrity, the involvement, the training and experience and the commitment of all concerned, and the objective must always be to guarantee the purity, reliability and reproductability of the medicines supplied to the practioners of the healing art.

High standards of personal cleanliness must be maintained by all personnel and hand washing facilities made available and used at regular intervals.

Protective clothing including gloves and hat should be worn in manufacturing facilities not only by the manufacturing personnel but also by the visitors. Cleanliness and proper hygienic conditions are the primary requirements. Utensils are required to be thoroughly washed after every use.

Incoming raw materials should be transferred to a quarantine store on each delivery. Each delivery is allocated a reference or batch number to identify the material in every stage of manufacture, samples are taken from every batch to carry out tests for raw material specifications. Specimens may be photographed in certain cases subjected to microstructure analysis from which micro photographs are taken. All raw materials are released from the quarantine store only after they are labeled as fit for use according to specifications. Rejected raw materials are stored separately for disposal. The finished products are packed and labeled subject to quality control inspections.

At every step of manufacturing all equipments are inspected to ensure that these are clean and free from all contaminations, all raw materials and equipments are carefully labeled to identify the material being processed and products are labeled at every stage with batch number, manufacturing procedure is strictly followed in each step of production and batch records are maintained indicating times, temperatures, weights, etc., so the history of every batch from raw materials used to labeling of finished products may be checked at a later date if necessary. at every step quality control personnel are required to make spot ch3eckings and collect samples for laboratrory analysis to ensure absolute quality control and thus purity of the products. On completion of manufacturing, representative samples of the products are taken and labelled with the batch number and identity. Analytical tests are carried out in the laboratory to ensure that the product meets the finished product specifications and thereafter the product is labelled as ready to despatch. Samples of each batch of the product is always retained in the laboratory. Storage conditions are carefully followed to ensure that the product does not deteriorate during transport or further storage at the stockists place.

General precautions for quality control include segregation of processing areas to avoid possible cross contamination, the use of laminar air flow equipment or air conditioners, and all operations including the segregation of processing areas to avoid any possible cross contamination, the use of laminar air flow or air conditioning and all operations are carried out in such a way that the risk of contamination is minimized. Microbiological testing by swab or settle plate method to monitor environmental contamination of the entire manufacturing area is recommended. Areas to be tested include laboratory benches water taps, valves and toilets.

Physical Properties

Spagyric Essences and Tinctures may be routinely tasted for their physical properties, including specific gravity, refractive index, colour, smell and taste.

General Tests

These may include plant residue(prior to burning), pH levels, water and alcohol content. Karl Fischer technique is the prescribed method for determining the water content.

Chemical Analysis

Conventions chemical methods are to be followed which could provide a means of identification and a guide of the purity to the spagyric tinctures, this include a thorough analysis for mineral salts and trace elements in the spagyric tinctures.

Thin Layer Chromatography

It utilizes the different migration rates for individual constituents of spagyric tinctures on a thin film of inert material. It shows characteristic bands on a layer of silica gel of 25-250 cm thickness, each band representing a specific chemical constituent of the spagyric tincture itself, but different batches of the same spagyric tincture. Various solvents are used such as butanol/acetic acid or methanol/chloroform over development distances of about 10 cm.It is used widely throughout the world in preparation of herbal tinctures to ascertain the purity, reproductivity and therapeutic effectiveness of the end products.

VEGA point testing or other types of analysis make it possible to determine and compare the amount of inherent energy in remedies produced by spagyric method. Here the huge qualitative advantages of spagyric remedies become obvious. Importantly, practitioners are able to experience the excellent efficacy of the spagyric medications through the fast, lasting results produced in patients. These remedies stimulate with their spagyric phyto-components, which provide an extra energy boost and regulate via the natural properties of individual plant constituents. This powerful combination creates "super-charged" remedies that invigorate the body's vital energy, act as immune system catalysts and promote more efficient cellular activity to help infected or weakened organ tissues resume normal function.

Kirlian Photography

In 1939, Semyon Kirlian discovered by accident that if an object on a photographic plate is subjected to a high-voltage electric field, an image is created on the plate. The image looks like a colored halo or coronal discharge. This image is said to be a physical manifestation of the spiritual aura or "life force" which allegedly surrounds each living thing.

Allegedly, this special method of "photographing" objects is a gateway to the world of auras. Actually, what is recorded is due to quite natural phenomena such as pressure, electrical grounding, humidity and temperature. Changes in moisture (which may reflect changes in emotions), barometric pressure, and voltage, among other things, will produce different 'auras'.

Living things are moist. When the electricity enters the living object, it produces an area of gas ionization around the photographed object, assuming moisture is present on the object. This moisture is transferred from the subject to the emulsion surface of the photographic film and causes an alternation of the electric charge pattern on the film. If a photograph is taken in a vacuum, where no ionized gas is present, no Kirlian image appears. If the Kirlian image were due to some paranormal fundamental living energy field, it should not disappear in a simple vacuum (Hines 2003).

There have even been claims of Kirlian photography being able to capture "phantom limbs," e.g., when a leaf is placed on the plate and then torn in half and "photographed," the whole leaf shows up in the picture. This is not due to paranormal forces, however, but to fraud or to residues left from the initial impression of the whole leaf.

Parapsychologist Thelma Moss popularized Kirlian photography as a diagnostic medical tool with her books The Body Electric (1979) and The Probability of the Impossible (1983). She was convinced that the Kirlian process was an open door to the "bioenergy" of the astral body. Moss came to UCLA in mid-life and earned a doctorate in psychology. She experimented with and praised the effects of LSD and was in and out of therapy for a variety of psychological problems, but managed to overcome her personal travails and become a professor at UCLA's Neuropsychiatric Institute. Her studies focused on paranormal topics, such as auras, levitation and ghosts. One of her favorite subjects at UCLA was Uri Geller, whom she "photographed" several times. She even made several trips to the Soviet Union to consult with her paranormal colleagues. Moss died in 1997 at the age of 78.

Moss paved the way for other parapsychologists to speculate that Kirlian "photography" was parapsychology's Rosetta stone. They would now be able to understand such things as acupuncture, chi, orgone energy, telepathy, etc., as well as diagnose and cure whatever ails us. For example, Bio-Electrography claims to be a method of investigation for biological objects, based on the interpretation of the corona-discharge image obtained during exposure to a high-frequency, high-voltage electromagnetic field which is recorded either on photo paper or by modern video recording equipment. Its main use is as a fast, inexpensive and relatively non-invasive means for the diagnostic evaluation of physiological and psychological states.

Kirlian photography (aka corona discharge photography or spark electrography) has been shown to demonstrate an electrochemical image of pre- and post-adjustment with definite change in image.

Research has been conducted in the former USSR, and in Germany, China, and the U.S., among other countries, which supports the use of Kirlian photography to measure or assess vital force in living systems, and to evaluate treatment methodology. Kirlian photography is a technique of photographing the electrical discharge from an object when impressed with a high voltage field. It was discovered by Semyon Kirlian in Russia in 1939. The Russians have performed scores of experiments on live plants, animals, and humans with the Kirlian effect. Kirov State University of Kazakhstan has studied the Kirlian effect with electron microscopy. Supposedly the Kirov scientists saw the living "double" of a living organism in motion. Kirlian photography is best remembered for revealing a leaf which, a portion of it having been cut away, revealed the entire leaf in terms of its aura. This is described as the phantom leaf effect. The Russians observed that the high-frequency discharge seems to imply the existence of an elementary plasma-like constellation made of ionized excited electrons, protons, and perhaps other particles and giving off its own electromagnetic fields and the basis of biological fields.1 In 1968, Drs. Inyushin, Grishchenko, Vorobev, Shouiski, Fedorova and Gibadulin announced that "all living things – plants, animals and humans not only have a physical body made of atoms and molecules but also a counterpart body of energy which they termed the Biological Plasma body."

Life force can be conceptualized through the energetic body model. Research with Kirlian photography has been performed by very reputable scientists. Its application to clinical sciences is still very much in its infancy. "Kirlian photography is considered safe but should not be used on people with pacemakers, heart disease, or during pregnancy".

The above discussion is to show that other healing arts and scientists have researched this technology. It is appropriate at this time that the Science of Plant Alchemy to look into this technology for future utilization especially to photograph the energy fields being transmitted by our medicines. Further serious study of this subject with research design methodology is encouraged.

22

Safety Measures in Laboratory

General Safety Rules:

1. Know the theory of the experiment we are considering. Do not attempt anything at random.
2. Study the properties of the products going to be produced or have to use in the production prior to the Experiment.
3. Operator's safety in the laboratory;

   Respect the safety regulation for gas, electricity etc,

   Never eat, drink or smoke in the laboratory.

   Always wear glasses.
4. Wear water proof rubber gloves which will protect us while handling acid or alkali liquids.
5. Wear asbestos gloves to handle molten liquids.
6. Wear asbestos gloves over the rubber gloves when handling acids or bases and hot liquids.
7. Wear leather or water- proof plastic shoes, no cloth or perforated shoes.
8. Have a working fire-extinguisher and a container filled with cold water close at hand. if there is an electrical heating system, make sure that the extinguisher is designed to extinguish electrical fires.
9. Mix unknown liquids in small quantity only. Always proceed as follows: pour a small amount of liquid in a test tube and a little bit of the other liquid into another test tube, close and keep the tubes away from each other. Mix the contents of the tubes slowly and must wear glasses when doing such kind of job.

10. Never pour a cold liquid in a hot liquid and vice versa.
11. Never pour water into an acid.
12. Permanent ventilation of the laboratory

    In case of the use of solvent

    In case of gas heating

    Fume hood for dangerous gases.

    No flames during work with volatile liquids.
13. The use of electrical heating is preferable during the handling of volatile liquids.
14. Never smell directly from a flask just wave a little.
15. Place wire gauze between the flask and the gas flame.
16. Never distill to dryness bodies giving peroxide, ether, acids etc. only water and alcohol can be distilled to dryness.
17. As much as possible, avoid any contact between rubber or cork stoppers and the extraction liquids.
18. Never force to join ground glass tubes.
19. Never exert mechanical force on glass welds.
20. Wet the flexible tubes (rubber or plastic) to be slipped on the glass.
21. Use cork or waxed- cork stoppers for distilled water or sulphur- free rubber stoppers.
22. Grease the ground joints silicon grease before joining. if a ground glass joint stick, try to pull the two parts apart, by hammering lightly on the ground joint with a plastic tool; if this too not work lightly heat the ground joint or use hot water.
23. To clean the glassware, rinse the flasks with ethyl alcohol, then with liquid detergent, followed with regular powder and then with clear water. Finish with a light rinse with distilled water or dematerialized water or dry the inside of the flask.
24. Bleach is excellent in all care, particularly to clean up calcinations residues. It must be less than three months old. Never bleach in contact with acid otherwise chlorine very toxic gas is given off.

23

Doctrine of Dosage

We treat acute diseases as a condition with sudden onset, clearly defined, severe symptoms and of relatively short duration. There may be some difference in opinion, as a general rule, these conditions are treated with low potencies at a high frequency of dosage (for instance, every half hourly, hourly etc.).

Chronic diseases are viewed as deep seated, probably inherited disease, with ill defined symptoms and time of onset of the diseases are long lasting, as a general rule, these conditions are treated with relatively high potencies at a low frequency of dosage (for instance, once a week, fortnightly etc.).

Arndt Schultz Law

Small doses encourage life, large doses impede life, very large doses destroy life. Drs. Bergeret and Tetau (of France) have explained the mode of action of medicines in the light of the current knowledge of immunology. Immunity is the protective mechanism of our body which is able to recognize and differentiate between useful and harmful elements having a cell or tissue memory, thus our body is equipped with an inbuilt mechanism to accept or reject any medicinal substances which are induced to effect a cure. Drs. Bergeret and Tetau also maintained that, Low potencies are stimulant, while they opined that, medium potencies are regulatory, and high potencies are depressant. Clinical research has demonstrated this principle, for instance, it has been observed that potencies of Folliculinum 9C depress folliculin secretion in female rats.

Dilutions in decimal scale are produced by adding one part of spagyric tincture with nine parts of distilled water/alcohol and labelled Ist dilution, successive dilutions are produced by adding one part of denominated dilution adding nine parts of distilled water/alcohol.

Recommended Dosage

Adults 10 drops

Children 5 drops

Dosage Frequency

Different reaction calls for different remedies

Generals than particulars

Improvement in condition times for decrease frequency of dosage

Condition cleared times for stop dosing

Excessive Aggravation times for stop dosing

New symptoms times for new remedy

Re-appearing symptoms times for repeatation of dosage of same remedy.

24

Medicinal Plants

Achillea millefolium

Common Names: MILFOIL, YARROW

Family: Compositae.

Habitats: Meadows and road side of Europe.

Part Used: Flower Clusters.

Indication: Anti-inflammatory, anti-septic, anti-spasmodic, arteriosclerosis to regulate the menstrual cycle, uterine, haemorrhages, to treat wounds, ulcer, sores furuncles, chilblains and cracks, chronic gastritis, hypochlorhydria, dyspepsia, liver malfunction.

Definition: Yarrow grows to 3 feet tall and has no branches except near the top. The leaves are alternate, 3-5 inches long, with many leaflets on each side of the midrib (1- pinnately lobed); and these are further divided into smaller leaflets, giving them a delicate, fernlike, lacy appearance. Flower heads are arranged in large, compact clusters at the top of the stem, each cluster consisting of 1 or more flower heads. The flower head has 20-25 yellowish-white (rarely pink) ray flowers and similarly colored disk flowers.

Description: *Achillea millefolium* is highly variable and has been treated both as a single species with varieties and as multiple distinct species. *A. millefolium* is cosmopolitan throughout the Northern Hemisphere. In North America, *A. millefolium* is a complex of both native and introduced plants and their hybrids.

Aconitum napellus

Common Name: MONKSHOOD

Family: Ranunculaceae.

Habitats: Europe and America.

Part Used: Root.

Indication: It is highly poisonous when plant reaches at maturity, chronic neuralgic pain especially, trigeminal nerve which affects the face sciatica nerve, to cure drug addication.

Definition: Plant with the high test concentrations of poison this concentration is only exceeded by an another species.

Description: Flower is beautiful, helmet shaped and may be darker blue, yellow or white in color, root is turnip shaped.

Constituents: Alkaloids (Aconite and Napelline); glycosides, resins, starch, manitol.

Adiantum capillus veneris

Common Names: VENUS HAIR, MAIDEN HAIR FERN

Family: Pteridaceae.

Habitats: Southern Europe, warm region of America.

Part Used: The tiny stems, leaves, peduncles.

Indication: For dry cough caused by irritation of upper respiratory tract, acute and chronic bronchitis, uterine, anti-spasmodic dymenorrhoea, strengthens hair.

Definition: the venus hair is one of the most used plants to strengthen and make hair grow, used in shampoos and cosmetics.

Description: Botanically it is fern whose sporangia are located in a fold of exterior boarder of the fronds (the leave like part of ferns) the stems and petioles are tiny smooth and bright. Leaves are slightly bitter, together with a faintly sweetish, aromatic, feebly astringent taste.

Constituents: Tannins, mucilage, sugar and essential oil.

Remark: Expectorant for chest catarrh, and the stems are used for hair wash.

Aesculus hippocastanum

Common Name: HORSE CHESTNUT

Family: Sapindaceae.

Habitats: Europe and America.

Part Used: Seeds and bark of young branches.

Indication: Stimulating effects on blood circulation, contains significant amounts of a coumarin glucoside called esculin. It has poisonous action on venous system and blood circulation, used in vericose vein in legs thrombophlebitis, haemorrhoids, prostate, used in cosmetics for soothing and protecting skin.

Definition: the fruit of this tree has a sour taste. Poisoning may occur if eaten in great amount.

Description: Leaves are high, palm shaped toothed and grow in many groups. Flowers are white and gather in clusters. Fruits are big, contain 1 or 2 seeds.

Constituents: Esculin, tannin, etheral oil, pectin, potash, calcium, phosphorus.

Agaricus muscarius

Common Name: TOADSTOOL

Family: Agaricaceae.

Habitats: Dry pine and birch forests in Europe, Asia and America.

Part Used: Fresh stips and pibus dried fungus.

Indication: Producing more vertigo and delirium followed by profound stupor with lowered reflexes.

Description: A very poisonous fungus grows all over the Northern Hemisphere in dry places and in summer. It is a rather attractive toadstool with bright red cap flecked with pale to dark orange marks.

Constituents: Muscarine, the poisonous alkaloid of Agaricus.

Ailanthus glandulosa

Common Name: CHINESE SUMACH/TREE OF GOD

Family: Simaroubaceae.

Habitats: China, Europe and Britain.

Part Used: Bark.

Indication: It has action on Gastro Intestinal Tract, also has anti-helminthic., anti-diarrheic and emetic properties.

Description: Tree growing to a height of about 65 feet with whitish lenticales. Flowers are calyx short cover lapping lobes, Gynaecium formed of carpels.

Constituents: Glycoside, resin, tannin and mucilage.

Allium cepa

Common Name: ONION

Family: Liliaceae.

Habitats: Native to Iran in Middle East, it is now widely spread and cultivated all over the world.

Part Used: Bulb.

Indications: Anti-biotic against skin infection, mucolytic and anti-inflammatory for expectorant and the pectoral, high blood pressure, obesity, rheumatism, kidney disease, chronic hepatitis, fatty degeneration of liver, cosmatics, stimulates hair grow, soothes and makes skin more beautiful clears skin from acne.

Description: growing up to one meter high during its first year of life it forms the bulb and during second year, the stem grows the plant blooms and renders fruit.

Constituents: Onion is rich in sulphured glycosides, plenty of enzymes, sulphur, iron, potassium, magnesium, fluorine, calcium, manganese and phosphorus, vitamins A, C and B complex.

Allium sativum

Common Name: GARLIC

Family: Amaryllidaceae.

Habitats: Asia, it is now cultivated worldwide.

Part Used: Bulb.

Indication: Raw, garlic extract, decoction of garlic cloves, oil and garlic sauce or emulsions are used in hypertension, hypotension, as blood thinner, hypolipidemic, hypoglycemic, anti-biotic and anti-septic, of diarrhoea, gastroenteritis and colitis, detoxification, prevents malignant growth, dyspepsia which cause flatulence, corn remover, expectorant, anti-asthmatic, specially anti-biotic for Salmonella, E-coli, Shigella, Staphylococcus.

Description: Vivacious plant of the Amaryllidaceae family, growing from 30-70 cm high, with whitish or reddish flowers. It's root has a bulb composed of several cloves.

Aloe capensis

Common Name: ALOE

Family: Asphodelaceae.

Habitats: America and Asia.

Part Used: Whole plant.

Indication: Bitter aloe is used as appetizer, stomachic and cholagogue. It has laxative, emmenagogue, purgative and oxytocic properties. It's juice is used in wounds, burns and other ailments of skin.

Description: growing up to 3-4 m high, it has fleshy, lanceolated, spiked leaves and red or yellow flowers.

Constituents: Polysaccharide, glycosides, enzymes and minerals.

Althaea officinalis

Common Name: ALTHAEA

Family: Malvaceae.

Habitats: Europe and America.

Part Used: Roots, leaves and flowers.

Indication: Laxative in constipation, anti-inflammatory in gastritis, colitis and gastroenteritis, digestive mucus membrane irritations, in children, when teeth are erupting.

Description: Sweetness and softness leaves are delicately covered with velvet like hairs and grows up to 2 m with large velvet like leaves and white flowers with 5 petals.

Infusion: 30 gm of young leaves or flowers or roots per lit of water. Drink three or four cups daily, sweetened with honey.

Constituents: Mucilage, pectin, mineral salts, vitamin-C.

Anthemis nobilis

Common Name: SWEET CHMOMILE, ROMAN CAMOMILE.

Family: Asteraceae.

Habitats: Europe, America.

Part Used: Flowers.

Indications: Anti-inflammatory, anti-spasmodic, used in gall bladder and liver colic, menstrual pain, compress is used in rheumatism, to heal wounds.

Description: Vivacious plant growing from 10-20 cm high. chamomile has finally divided leaves and flowers which are quite similar to german chamomile.

Constituents: Etheral oil, isobutyric acid, inositol, methyl crotonic acid glucosides anthemic acids, free fatty acid, anthosterol.

Arnica montana

Common Name: ARNICA

Family: Asteraceae.

Habitats: Europe, North and South America.

Part Used: Flowers and root.

Indications: If use internally, it is highly poisonous to nervous system, used for skin as anti-inflammatory, bruises, sprain, hematomas, used for furuncles, abscess.

Description: The plant is 30-50 cm high, with composed flowers, bright yellow in color, very exuberant. It can be easily mistaken with Inula, whose medicinal properties have not been exhaustively studied, unlike these false Arnica true Arnica has only 1-2 pairs of leaves, which grows in opposite pairs.

Constituents: Essential oil, phenolic substances, flavonoids and tannin.

Artemisia abrotanum

Common Name: SOUTHERN WOOD

Family: Asteraceae.

Habitats: South East Europe, West Asia.

Part Used: leaves and stems.

Indications: Insomnia, skin ailments, leaf tea is tonic and dispel parasitic worms from children. It is rubbed on the skin to deter flies and placed among cloth to repel moths.

Description: It is strongly aromatic, shrubby perennial, it has semi green thread like leaves and small dense head of yellow florets which appear in summer.

Constituents: Abrotannin, tannin, essential oil.

Artemisia cina

Common Name: WORM SEED

Family: Asteraceae.

Habitats: North Africa, Eurasia.

Part Used: Flowers, leaves, shoot.

Indication: It's infusion is useful for complaints of the nervous system and the digestive tract, also used as a febrifuge , the seed contain the vermicide "santonin" which is an effective and rapid treatment for round worms, it is also effective for thread worms, it is poisonous in large doses.

Description: This fast growing pungent perennial plant has deeply indented foliage covered in fine hair and small, round, yellow flowers head.

Constituents: Two crystalline sesquiterpene lactones, santonin and artemisin and a volatile oil.

Atropa belladonna

Common Name: DEADLY NIGHT SHADE

Family: Solanaceae.

Habitats: Southern and Central Europe and South America.

Part Used: Leaves and root.

Indication: Used to treat a number of conditions, including irritable bowel syndrome, spastic colon, stomach ulcers, parkinson's disease, diverticulitis, motion sickness, excessive night time urination, pink eyes.

Description: It's most common name, belladonna, derives from Italian, meaning "beautiful woman." Historically, women have used the herb's oil to dilate and enlarge the pupils for seductive effect. It is a branching plant that often grows to resemble a shrub of about 4 feet in height within a single growing season. Its leaves are long, extending 7 inches, and its bell-shaped flowers are purple with green tinges, about an inch long. The fruit and berries appear green when growing, but, as the toxins get stronger in the ripening stage, turn a shiny black color.

Constituents: Hyoscyamine, atropine, atropamine, belladonnine and hyoscine.

Avena sativa

Common Name: OATS

Family: Poaceae.

Habitats: Europe, cultivated around the temperate world.

Part Used: Seeds and leaves.

Indication: Influences the nutritive functions of brain and the nervous system, a mild and gentle aphrodisiac. Nervous exhaustion, nerve tremors of the aged; chorea, paralysis agitans, epilepsy. Post-diphtheritic paralysis, rheumatism of heart, colds, insomnia. Oats are also used in external preparations to treat eczema and dry skin.

Description: An annual with erect culms (stems) 40–180 cm long. Its leaves are cauline. The spikelets consist of 2 or 3 fertile florets, and are wedge-shaped, laterally compressed, 22–27 mm long and persistent on the plant.

Chemical Constituents: Minerals, lipids, ß-glucan, a mixed-linkage polysaccharide, phytoconstituents like avenanthramides, an indole alkaloid-gramine, flavonoids, flavonolignans, triterpenoid saponins, sterols, and tocols.

Berberis vulgaris

Common Name: BARBERRY

Family: Berberidaceae.

Habitats: Europe and America.

Part Used: Bark, Root.

Indication: Cholagogue and Digestive, Laxative, Heart and circulatory invigorating, diuretic and febrifuge.

Description: It is an erect deciduous shrub, from three to eight feet high, with leaves of an obviate-oval form, terminated by soft bristles, about two inches long, and one-third as wide. The flowers are small and yellow in clusters, and the fruit bright-red oblong berries, in branches, and tastes sour.

Constituents: Glucose, levulose, vitamin-c, citric and malic acid.

Betula alba

Common Name: BIRCH TREE, WHITE BIRCH

Family: Betulaceae.

Habitats: Europe, Canada, America.

Part Used: Leaves, Buds and Bark.

Indication: Used for edema, premenstrual syndrome, kidney calculus, depurative skin afflictions, decoction is used to decrease fever, compress is used for wounds and sores.

Description: A deciduous, soft wood slender tree which grows to a height of 100 feet or more.

Leaves: Dark green above, light green below.

Constituents: Betulin, betulinic acid, betuls camphor, flavonoids, tannin and essential oil.

Cannabis sativa

Common Name: HEMP

Family: Cannabaceae.

Habitats: Asia.

Part Used: Flowers and Fruits.

Indication: Neuralgic and rheumatic pain.

Description: Plant grow up to 1.5 meter high, leaves are palm shaped, divided in to 5-6 segment with a toothed edge.the flowers are greenish and appear in terminal bouquets.

Constituents: Cannabinol, cannibidiol, choline, trigonelline acid.

Capsella bursa pastoris

Common Name: SHEPHERD'S PURSE

Family: Brassicaceae.

Habitats: Grows worldwide.

Part Used: Whole Plant.

Indication: Haemostatic, oxytocic, infusion is used for uterine hemorrhages, labour acceleration, intestinal atony, low blood pressure, epistaxis, compress is used for skin wound and bleeding.

Description: Annual plant grow up to 50 cm high. Its leaves grow in the from of a rose, near the soil and it has small, white flowers. The fruits are triangle-shaped.

Constituents: Choline, acetylcholine, malic acid, citric acid, saponin, potassium, tannin.

Carduss benedictus

Common Name: BENEDICTINE, HOLY THISTLE

Family: Asteraceae.

Habitats: Asia.

Part Used: Leaves, flowers, stem, seeds, roots.

Indication: To purify and strengthen circulation, small doses treat digestive problems and infections, expel catarrh and applied on wound.

Description: An annual herb, grows about 2 feet high, is reddish, slender, very much branched, leaves are long, narrow, clasping the dull green stem, with prominent pale veins, the irregular teeth of the wavy margin ending in spines. The flowers are pale yellow, in green prickly heads, each scale of the involucre, or covering of the head, ending also in a long, brown bristle.

Constituents: The herb contains B-complex vitamins, calcium, iron and manganese.

Caulophyllum thalictroides

Common Name: BLUE COHOSH

Family: Berberidaceae.

Habitats: America, Asia.

Part Used: Whole plant.

Indication: It is used for stimulating the uterus and starting labor; starting menstruation; stopping muscle spasms; as a laxative; and for treating colic, sore throat, cramps, hiccups, epilepsy, hysterics, inflammation of the uterus, and joint conditions.

Description: Leaves are alternate, flowers are bisexual, which produces rhizomes, brownish grey about 4 inches long. Roots are tough and of pale brown color.

Constituents: Bitter principal and saponins.

Cetraria islandica

Common Name: ICELAND MOSS

Family: Parmeliaceae.

Habitats: Europe and America.

Part Used: Dried thallus.

Indication: Anti-biotic, anti-emetic, appetizer, demulcent, disinfectant, galactogogue, nutritive and tonic.

Description: It is a lichen growing to 0.1 m by 0.5 m at a slow rate with light brown stem deeply divided into unequal lobules.

Constituents: Sugar, gum, mucilage, lichen starch, potassium, iron, sodium, magnesium.

Chelidonium majus

Common Name: CELANDINE

Family: Papaveraceae.

Habitats: Europe and North America.

Part Used: Leaves, roots.

Indication: Nephritis, asthma, angina pectoris, biliary colic, jaundice and liver insufficiency, also used for warts, herpes, and callus.

Definition: It is a brittle, herbaceous biennial that reaches 30-80 cm in height. Its stems are ribbed and branching. The lower parts of the branches are pubescent. When the branches or leaves are broken a yellowish-orange sap can be seen. Flowers are yellow having fetid odour.

Description: a plant of the poppy family, commonly known as greater celandine.

Constituents: Alkaloids, chelidonine chelerythrin, homochelidonine A, homocheli donine B. Chelerythrin is narcotic and poisonous. Also, protopine and sanguinarine, and chelidoxanthin, a bitter principle.

Chenopodium anthelmintic

Common Names: JERUSALUM OAK, WORM SEED

Family: Chenopodiacease.

Habitats: America, Europe.

Part Used: Leaves, flowers.

Indication: Stomachic invigorator and carminative, anti-helminthic and vermifuge.

Definition: People used worm seed because of its medicinal properties, its leaves and flowers have a strong aroma due to essential oil.

Description: It grows from 40-100 cm in height with branched stems and yellowish or greenish small flowers.

Constituents: Alkaloids, anthraquinones, flavonoids, saponins, tanins, sterols, reducing sugars, glycosides, resins, triterpenes, proteins and coumarins.

Cimcifuga racemosa

Common Names: BLACK COHOSH, BLACK SNAKEROOT

Family: Ranunculaceae.

Habitats: America.

Part Used: Fresh root.

Indication: Menopausal symptoms, premenstrual syndrome (PMS), painful menstruation, acne, weakened bones (osteoporosis), and for starting labor in pregnant women., headache, cough, asthma.

Description: A large herbaceous perennial wildflower bush like plant, 3-6 ft tall, with compound, toothed leaves and long candles of tiny, white, fuzzy flowers.

Constituents: Triterpene glycosides, phenolic acids, flavonoids, volatile oils, and tannins.

Cinchona calisaya

Common Name: YELLOW BARK

Family: Rubiaceae.

Habitats: West Indies, Australia, Africa.

Part Used: Bark, root.

Indication: Febrifuge, appetizer, also used for loss of hair.

Description: Peruvian shrub or small tree having large glossy leaves and cymes of fragrant yellow to green or red flowers.

Constituents: Quinine, quinidine, cinchonine, cinhonidinc.

Cinchona succirubra

Common Name: RED BARK

Family: Rubiaceae.

Habitats: West Indies, Australia, Africa.

Part Used: Bark, root.

Indications: Febrifuge, appetizer, also used for loss of hair.

Description: A tree said to reach 50-80 feet in height, leaves are pubescent petioles, flat above; stipules oblong, obtuse, dark green and shining above, much paler and finely pubescent on the leaves beneath. Inflorescence and flowers as in the other species. Fruit variable in form. Seeds as in the other species.

Constituents: Quinine, quinidine, cinchonine, cinhonidinc.

Clematis erecta

Common Names: VIRGIN BONER, TRAVELLER'S JOY

Family: Ranunculaceae.

Habitats: Europe, Iran, Afghanistan.

Part Used: Flower, leaves, stem.

Indications: Analgesic, leaves are used as diuretic also as ointment for pain relief blister, sores and inflmmation.

Description: This deciduous, scrambling, semi woody, climber has oval leaflets and fragnants greenish white flowers.

Constituents: Anemonin, diacrylic acid, saponin and essential oil.

Cochlearia officinalis

Common Name: SCURVY GRASS

Family: Brassicaceae.

Habitats: Europe, America.

Part Used: Whole plant.

Indications: Anti-scorbutic, appetizer and digestive, diuretic and depurative, rubefacient that acts on the blood towards the skin thus reducing the congestion of internal organs.

Definition: The scurvy grass is still used due to its medicinal properties and fine odour.

Constituents: Vitamin C. Leaves abound in a pungent oil containing sulphur of the butylic series.

Condurango marsdenia

Common Names: CUNDURANGO, CONDOR PLANT

Family: Apocynaceae and Asclepiadaceae.

Habitats: Colombia, Africa, Asia, America.

Part Used: Fruits.

Indications: Used in gastric debility, especially relieves pain in the stomach. It acts upon the central nervous system, producing impairment of appetite, vomiting, ptyalism, muscular weakness, convulsions and paralysis.

Description: This vine plant grows from 30-125 cm in height, having opposite cordate leaves, hairy above and silky and tomentose underneath. The flowers are borne in loose cymes. The peduncles and petioles are covered with a pale, grayish pubescence, and the stem, bark has a greenish-gray color, which exudes a viscid, milky juice.

Constituents: Condurangin, conduransterin, cinnamic acid, resin, gum, glucose, tannin, cellulose, lignin and alkaloids etc.

Conium maculatum

Common Names: HEMLOCK, POISON HEMLOCK

Family: Umbelliferea.

Habitats: Europe and America.

Part Used: Fruits.

Indications: To relieve nervous excitation and give rest; neuralgic or rheumatic pains in the old and feeble, or where there are caco-plastic deposits, pain in stomach, pain of gastric ulcer, nervousness and restlessness.

Description: It grows from 30-125 cm high, erect, round, hollow, glaucous, copiously spotted and dotted with dull purple. The leaves are tripinnate; pinnate, bright-green, leaflets are ovate, lanceolate flowers are small, white, all fertile, petals are obcordate, 5 in number. The fruit roundish-ovate, of a pale-green color. The whole plant exhales a disagreeable, virose odor.

Constituents: Conicine and cicutine, conhydrine, pseudo-conhydrine, methyl-conine and ethyl-piperidine, gum, resin and alkaloids.

Daphne mezereum

Common Names: MEZEREON, SPURGE OLIVE

Family: Thymelaeaceae.

Habitats: East Himalayas.

Part Used: Bark, flowers, leaves, root seed.

Indication: Used as anti-septic, applied on small cuts, to treat fever, intestinal problem, toxic seeds expel worms.

Description: It is evergreen shrub with cluster of fragrant, white to pink flowers and small dark berries.

Constituents: Mezeen, daphnin, mezereic acid, a greenish brown amorphous resin, glycosides, mucilage, oil, wax, a euphorbone like substance.

Dictamnus albus

Common Names: BURNING BUSH, DITTANY

Family: Rutaceae.

Habitats: Europe.

Part Used: Leaves, root and bark.

Indication: Used as emmenagogue, digestive, anti-spasmodic, vermifuge, invigorating diuretic.

Definition: a genus of flowering plant with a single species, it has several geographical variants. It is also known as candel plant, gas plant, and fraxinella.

Description: Growing from 50-60 cm in height with leaves resembling those of a bird's tongue and large, aromatic, white or pink flowers.

Constituents: Alkaloids, limonoid triterpenoids, flavonoids, sesquiterpenoids, coumarins, and phenylpropane.

Drosera rotundifolia

Common Name: SUNDEW

Family: Droseraceae.

Habitats: America.

Part Used: Aerial parts of the plant.

Indications: Anti-tussive, antibiotic, anti-spasmodic, acute and chronic bronchitis.

Description: A typical sundew plant with a diameter of around 3-5 cm, with a 5–25 cm tall inflorescence. The flowers grow on one side of a single slender, hairless stalk that emanates from the centre of the leaf rosette. White or pink in colour, the five-petalled flowers produce 1.0–1.5 mm, light brown, slender, tapered seeds.

Constituents: Acrid resin, sponin, napthoquinone, glucose, propionic acid, droserin.

Echinacea angustifolia

Common Names: ECHINACEA, CONE FLOWERS

Family: Asteraceae.

Habitats: America and Europe.

Part Used: Root.

Indication: Antibiotic effect on several germs, kills bacteria and fungi, immunostimulant, anti-inflamatory, anti-toxic and anti-viral, anti-cancerous, influenza, sinussitis, tonsillitis, acute and chronic respiratory infection, snake and insects bites.

Description: plants whose hollow stem grow up to one meter high. it has elongated, hairy, narrow leaves and mauve flower which grow on the tip of the stems and are quite exuberant.

Constituents: Polyacetylenes and polyenes, terpenes, pinene, thiyone.

Equisetum arvense

Common Name: HORSE TAIL

Family: Equisetaceae.

Habitats: Europe and America.

Part Used: Sterile stem and their branches.

Indications: Degenerative process of the skin, conjunctive tissue, fragile nail, breast flaccidity, arthrosis, ulceration, abscesses, infected wounds, eczema, osteoporosis, bone breaking, arteriosclerosis, oedema, urinary infection.

Definition: It is a perennial plant produces fertile and infertile shoots that are deciduous, by spores rather than seeds.

Description: The stems are erect and usually bear many branches in whorls. There are conspicuous sheaths at the nodes, above the whorled branches.

Constituents: The plant contains silica and silicic acids, a saponin called equisetonin, the flavone glycosides isoquercitrin, equisetrin, and galuteolin, also contains beta-sitosterol, campestrol, isofucosterol, and trace amounts of cholesterol, bioflavonoids, as well as manganese, potassium, sulfur and magnesium.

Ervum lens

Common Name: LENTIL

Family: Fabaceae.

Habitats: South-West Europe, Bengal, Rajasthan.

Part Used: Seeds.

Indication: Anti-inflammatory, helps prevent heart diseases, helps lower levels of homocysteine, an amino acid that is an intermediate product of an important metabolic process called the methylation cycle. The methylation cycle plays an important role in many processes like detoxification and brain function. Magnesium improves the flow of blood, oxygen and nutrients throughout the body, reduces cholesterol and soothes gastric troubles and constipation.

Description: A slender herb of height upto 8 in, leaves are small pointed, flowers purple blue. Seeds are lenticular, of various colours and sizes.

Constituents: Globulin, fiber, protein, folate and magnesium.

Erythraea centaurium

Common Name: CENTURY

Family: Gentianaceae.

Habitats: Britain, Europe, Western Asia.

Part Used: Leaves.

Indication: It is appetizer, aromatic, bitter, cholagogue, diaphoretic, digestive, emetic, weakly febrifuge, hepatic, stomachic and tonic, acts on the liver and kidneys, purifies the blood and is an excellent tonic for the digestive system.

Description: It is a annual/biennial growing to 0.3 m by 0.2 m. Leaves are elliptical. It flowers from June to October, flowers are pink, and the seeds ripen from August to October, 1-20 in long.

Constituents: Phenolic acids, sterols, glycosides, flavonoids, fatty acids, alkenes, waxes, resins, and essential oil.

Eucalyptus globulus

Common Name: BLUE GUM TREE

Family: Myrtaceae.

Habitats: Europe, America, Asia.

Part Used: Leaves and woods.

Indication: Bronchial catarrh, asthma, acute and chronic bronchitis, colitis, diarrhoea, intestinal fermentation.

Description: Tall tree growing up to 100 mt high, it has smooth, light colored trunk and evergreen spear shaped leaves.

Constituents: Aldehydes, a terpene and p-cymene, essential oil, tannin, eucalyptol.

Evonymus europaeus

Common Name: SPINDLE TREE

Family: Celastraceae.

Habitats: Europe, Western Asia, Britain.

Part Used: Seeds, fruit and barks.

Indication: Acts on the liver, tonic, alterative, cholagogue, laxative and hepatic stimulant.

Description: It is a deciduous shrub growing to 6 m, leaves are pointed, opposite, bark smooth, grey in color, occur in curved pieces. Flowers are bisexual or unisexual, appear in May or June in small groups, fruits-round, 4 lobed fleshy capsule from May to June and the seeds ripen from September to November.

Constituents: A bitter principle, a resin called euonymin, euonic acid, a crystalline glucoside, asparagin, resins, fat and dulcitol.

Euphorbium officinalis

Common Name: SPURGE

Family: Euphorbiaceae.

Habitat: India.

Part Used: Dry latex (Gum Resin).

Indications: Breathing disorders including asthma, bronchitis and chest congestion. It is also used for mucus in the nose and throat, throat spasms, hay fever, and tumors. Some people use it to cause vomiting. Indians used it for treating worms, severe diarrhea (dysentery), gonorrhea, and digestive problems.

Description: A perennial species, flowers are whitish, minute. Fruits are small, 1-2 mm in diameter, stems are round, erect, covered with yellow hair leaves.

Chemical Constituents: Euphorbone, a resin called euphorbo, euphorbic acid, calcium malate (25 per cent.), an intensely acrid substance.

Euphrasia officinalis

Common Name: EYE BRIGHT

Family: Orobanchaceae.

Habitats: Europe.

Part Used: Flowers, leaves and shoot.

Indication: Used as eye tonic, treating strain and infection, antiseptic, astringent, anti-inflammatory, having catarrh reducing properties ease the irritation in the eyes and running nose of hay fever and sinusitis.

Description: A annual herb grows two to eight inches tall with deep cut leaves and white or purple blooms that have yellow variegations. There are opposite branches on an erect stem with leaves that will be up to 1/2 an inch long. Flowers are on terminal spokes with a two-lipped corolla.

Constituents: Iridoid glycosides, flavonoids, quercetin, apigenin, and tannins. The most studied constituent of eyebright is aucubin and its aglycone, aucubigenin.

Fucus vesiculosus

Common Names: SEA WARE, SEA KELP

Family: Fucaceae.

Habitats: Europe.

Part Used: The thallus.

Indication: Acidity, oesophagic reflex, hiatus hernia, pyrosis, nourshing, remineralizing, anti-scury, mild laxative, hyperthyroidism, poultices are use in cellulitis, wrinkle, skin flaccidity.

Definition: Algae are water plant with chlorophyll or other coloring substances, whose size vary from microorganism to the size of an earth planet.

Description: This plant is brown in color, it's thallus is formed by tape shaped sheets which stick by their base to under water rocks, the reproductive system of the algae is located in its apex.

Constituents: It contains iodine, calcium, magnesium, potassium, sodium, phenolics, phloroglucinol, fucophorethols, phlorotannins, mucopolysaccharides, algin, lipids, and diglycerides.

Galeopsis ochroleuca

Common Name: HEMP NETTLE

Family: Lamiaceae.

Habitat: West Europe, including Britain, from Denmark to Germany and Spain.

Part Used: Leaves.

Indication: It is astringent, diuretic and mildly expectorant, used for whooping cough, bronchitis, tracheitis, disorders of the spleen.

Description: It is an annual growing upto 0.6 m (2ft). It is in flower from July to October. The flowers are hermaphrodite (have both male and female organs) and are pollinated by Bees. The plant is self-fertile. Flowers are white and yellowish in color.

Constituents: a tannin, silicates, iridoids, acetylharpagide, antirrhinoside, glucoside.

Genista scoparius (Tinctoria)

Common Name: DYER'S GREEN WOOD

Family: Fabaceae.

Habitats: Native to Mediterranean region, Canary Islands, Western Asia, Britain. It is found in meadows and pastures in Europe and Turkey. Established in the United States.

Part Used: Flower, leaves, bark, seed.

Indication: Flowering tops are used as dye and added to wood dyed blue cloth to turn it kendal green, used to treat tumors, rheumatism, diuretics, purative and weak cardio active properties.

Description: It is a shrub with golden flowers and small fruit pods with 4-10 seed.

Constituents: Scopnarine, yellow crystals, sparteine, tannin, sugar, essential oil.

Gentiana lutea

Common Name: YELLOW GENTIAN, GENTIAN

Family: Gentianaceae.

Habitats: Europe, and America.

Part Used: Root.

Indication: Chronic gastritis with lack of gastric juice, indigestion, vomiting, lack of appetite, liver congestion and biliary dysfunction.

Description: It grows 60-100 cm high with smooth upright stem which is large oval.

Constituents: Gentiopicrin, amarogenin, amaroswerin, gentiosid and gentinin, which is a mixture of gentiopicrin and gentinin. It also contains a flavonoid alkaloid commonly known as gentisin (Syn: Gentianic acid, Gentianin, Gentin), tannin, sugar, essential oil.

Glechoma hederacea

Common Name: GROUND IVY

Family: Lamiaceae.

Habitats: Europe and America.

Part Used: Flower.

Indication: Expectorant and pectoral for chronic bronchitis, wounds, hemorrhoids.

Description: An aromatic, perennial, evergreen creeper. It has ground stems, growing upto 25 cm in height. Flowers usually appear in clusters of three in the axils, in the area between the stem and petiole. Flowers are blue-violet, 3/8 to 5/16 in long.

Constituents: Essential oil, choline, tannin and phenolic acid.

Guaiacum officinale

Common Names: LIGNUM VITAE, GUAIAC WOOD

Family: Zygophyllaceae.

Habitat: America, Mexico, Colombia, Venezuela and West Indies.

Part Used: Gum resin of wood and bark.

Indication: Balsamic and expectorant, diuretic, sudorific and depurative for rheumatism, arthritis, gout, hypertension, arteriosclerosis, syphilis.

Definition: Guaiacum officinale is a slow growing, small to medium sized tree. The trunk is short and seldom straight, covered with a smooth, mottled, gray-green bark and topped with a dense crown of dark green leaves.

Description: Growing up to 10 m high with a trunk diameter of 60 cm. yellowish in color, very hard, resinous wood, compound leaves with follicles and small flowers.

Hamamelis virginiana

Common Name: WITCH HAZAL

Family: Hamamelidaceae.

Habitats: United States, Canada and Europe.

Part Used: Leaves and bark.

Indication: Dry extract and infusion use venotonic for varicose venis, phlebitis and hemorrhoids, hemostatic metorrhagias and menopausal disorder, compress is used for skin to activate blood flow also for dermatitis dry skin to eye washing use for eye sedatives.

Definition: The fruits of this tree are woody capsules similar to hazelnuts and when ripe they explode noisily at present the hazels is one of the most effective plants known to fight circulatory affection.

Description: Growing up to few meters high alternate oval shaped leaves and yellow flower of four tongue-shaped petals.

Constituents: Tannins, bitter principles, catechins, gallotannins, hamamelitannins, flavonoids (quercetin, kaempferol), phenolic acids, saponins and safrole, hamemeli, tannin, oxalate, calcium, gallic acid.

Humulus lupulus

Common Name: HOPS

Family: Cannabaceae.

Habitats: Europe and America.

Part Used: Flowers and fruits.

Indication: Nervous states, insomnia, migraine, sexual hyperexciation, dysphasia, lack of appetite, for herbal breast enlargement.

Definition: Hops is a plant that grows on bines; long stout stems with strong hairs to aid climbing that can reach 22 ft in height.

Constituents: Linalool, amino acid, asparagin, poly-phenolic tannin and resin.

Hydrastis canadensis

Common Name: GOLDEN SEAL.

Family: Ranunculaceae.

Habitat: Europe and America.

Part Used: Rhizome.

Properties: Anti-septic, anti-inflamatory, excessive menstruation and leucorrhoea, conjunctivitis.

Definition: A North American perennial herb in the buttercup family, having small greenish-white flowers and a yellow root used in herbal medicine.

Description: Growing from 20 cm high, its stems grow from an underground root, large palm shaped, leaves are dark green.

Constituents: Isoquinoline alkaloids: hydrastine, berberine, berberastine, hydrastinine, tetrahydroberberastine, canadine, and canalidine.

Hyoscyamus niger

Common Name: HENBANE

Family: Solanceae.

Habitat: Central Europe and America.

Part Used: Leaves.

Indication: Anti-spasmodic, analgesic and narcotic, used in asthma, toothache, ointment is used for rheumatism, gout.

Definition: Henbane is a poisonous plant that originated in Eurasia, though it is now globally distributed.

Description: High of up to one meter. It's flowers are pale yellow covered with a net of thin violet capillaries.

Constituents: Hyoscyamine, salt, gum, atropine, scopolamine, starch and volatile oil.

Imperatoria ostruthium

Common Name: HOGFENNEL, MASTER WORT

Family: Umbelliferae.

Habitat: Central and Southern Europe.

Part Used: Root and Seeds.

Indication: Anti-spasmodic, carminative, emmenagogic.

Description: It is a perennial growing to 1.2 m. It is dense, shrubby, with protruding flower stalks, stem erect, branched, hollow leaves bitripinnatified, basal leaves sheathed, it is in flower from June to August. Root is blackish.

Constituents: It contents coumarins, including oxypeucedanin, ostruthol, imperatorin, osthole, isoimperatorin and ostruthin.

Ledum palustre

Common Name: MARSH TEA

Family: Ericaceae.

Habitat: Europe and America.

Part Used: Leaves.

Indication: Diuretics, anti-cough external application for itching.

Description: It is a shrub 1-3 feet high, stems are erect, shruby, slender leaves, alternate and sessile.

Constituents: Ascaridole, p-cymene, myrtenal, hydrocarbons, ketones, monoterpenes, sesquiterpenes, flavonoids and essential oils.

Lobelia inflata

Common Name: INDIAN TOBACOO (GLANT LOBELIA)

Family: Campanulaceae.

Habitats: North America.

Part Used: Whole plant.

Indication: Anti-Emetic, anti-asthmatic, diaphoretic, expectorant and sedative.

Description: Its stem is 20 in high erect and angular, leaves are alternate, flowers are pale blue, fruits are swollen and dark brown.

Constituents: It contains apigenin, lobeline, lobelanine, isolobelanine, lobelanidine, quercetin, coumarins, glucosides, flavonoids, gum, resin, fixed oil, salts of lime and potassium, with ferric oxide.

Lycopodium clavatum

Common Name: CLUB MOSS, STAG'S HORN

Family: Lycopodiaceae.

Habitats: Europe and north America.

Part Used: Spores.

Indication: Gastric and urinary disorder, antipruritic, decongestant, diuretic and stomachic, anti-spasmodic, sedative, used for wounds and eczema.

Description: This toxic, evergreen, moss like herb has trailing stems, upright branches and developing ripe spores.

Constituents: It contains vanillic, coumaric, ferulic acids and syringic acids, huperzine A, lycopodine, lycoflexine, Alpha-onocerin, sporopollenin, polyphenol, alkaloids lycopodine, clavatine and clavatoxine; polyphenolic acids, including dihydrocaffeic and triterpenes.

Malva sylvestris

Common Names: MALLOW, MUSK MALLOW

Family: Malvaceae.

Habitats: Europe and America.

Part Used: Flowers, leaves, shoot, root.

Indication: It contain vitamins A, B, C, used for soothing skin, also as cough syrup.

Description: It has faintly musky, elegantly cut and round shallow lobed leaves with large white and pink flowers.

Constituents: It contains malvin and malonylmalvin. It also contains the naphtoquinone, malvone, ephedrine, pseudoephedrine, phytosterol, potassium nitrate and alkaloids, mucilage, malvine, malvidine, tannin.

Matricaria chamomilla

Common Name: GERMAN CHAMOMILLA

Family: Asteraceae.

Habitats: Europe and Asia.

Part Used: Flowers.

Indication: It is used topically in skin and mucous membrane inflammations and skin diseases, GI spasms and inflammatory diseases.

Description: It has fine foliage and honey daisy flowers with white petals and conical centers, blue, yellow or white in color, root is turnip shaped.

Constituents: It contains terpene bisabolol, farnesene, chamazulene, flavonoids (including apigenin, quercetin, patuletin and luteolin) and coumarin.

Melissa officinalis

Common Names: BALM, LEMON BALM

Family: Lamiaceae.

Habitats: Southern Europe and America.

Part Used: Leaves and flowers.

Indication: Anti-spasmodic, anti-septic, sedative, carminative, stress and depression, insomnia, menstrual pain, anti-fungal and anti-viral.

Definition: is a bushy herbaceous perennial of the mint family. Leaves are edible and may be added to salads, soups, sauces or vegetables. Leaves are also used to flavor teas.

Description: Grows up to 30-70 cm high. Wrinkled, ovate, medium green leaves (to 3" long) appear in pairs on square stems rising to 2' tall. Tiny, two-lipped, white flowers appear in the leaf axils throughout summer.

Constituents: It contain rosmarinic acid, caffeic acids, chlorogenic acid, and metrilic acid, tannins, flavonoids, and volatile oils, including citronellal, citral a (geranial), citral b (neral), methyl citronellate, ocimene, citronellol, geraniol, nerol, ß-caryophyllene, ß-caryophyllene oxide, linalool, and ethric oil.

Menyanthes trifoliata

Common Names: BUCK BEAN, BOGBEAN.

Family: Menyanthaceae.

Habitats: Europe and America.

Part Used: Flowers, leaves, root.

Indication: Used as a tonic to cleanse the blood, stimulate appetite, rheumatic pain, irregular menstruation.

Constituents: Melyanthine, choline, gum, saponin and tannin.

Myrtus communis

Common Names: MYRTLE, SWEET MYRTLE

Family: Myrtaceae.

Habitats: North Africa.

Part Used: Flowers, leaves, fruit nuts.

Indication: Used for digestive, respiratory and urinary problems, have antibacterial, analgesic and strong anti-inflammatory properties also have a highly selective cytostatic effect on tumours.

Description: It is an evergreen shrub or small tree, growing to 5 m tall. The leaf is entire, 3–5 cm long, with a fragrant essential oil. The star-like white flower has five petals and sepals, the fruit is a berry blue-black or yellow-amber in colour.

Constituents: Myrtenol, myrtol, aldehydes, resin, tannin.

Nasturtium officinalis

Common Name: WATER CRESS

Family: Brassicaceae.

Habitat: Europe and America.

Part Used: Flowers, leaves, stem.

Indication: It is a good source of lutein and beta-carotene, two important components in preventing UV-damage and maintaining skin health, which is key to an anti-ageing regime. It may also help in treating eczema, acne, and generally problematic skin.

The antioxidant properties of watercress especially help in preventing the damage to cells caused by smoking, thus potentially helping lower the cancer risk for lung and throat cancers.

Description: This aquatic herb has pungent, compound leaves and small white flowers in spring and summer.

Constituents: Vitamins A, B, C and E, nicotinamide, a glycoside, gluconasturtin, volatile oil, manganese, iron, phosphorus, potassium, iodine, copper, calcium, glycosides, protein, omega-3 fatty acids, antioxidants, leucine, fibre and sulphur.

Oxalis acetosella

Common Name: WOOD SORREL

Family: Oxalidaceae.

Habitat: Europe and America.

Part Used: Flowers, leaves and root.

Indication: Astringent and diuretic, used to treat fever and urinary problems, used to remove cancerous growth from lips and external wash for rashes and boils.

Description: Leaves are divided into fine segments, it has crepping rhizome, trifoliate leaves and white flowers, the leaves and flowers droop at night.

Constituents: Potassium binoxalate, ascorbic acid, mucilage.

Petroselinum sativum

Common Name: PARSLEY

Family: Umbelliferae.

Habitats: South Europe.

Part Used: Leaves, root, stems, seeds.

Indication: Emmenagogue, tonic, diuretic, aperient, abortifacient reduces the release of tamine, relieves rheumatism, tones uterine muscles after birth, soothes sprain and cuts.

Description: It is a biennial plant has a fleshy, spindle-shaped root, and an erect, smooth, branching stem. The radical leaves are biternate, bright green, and on long petioles; leaflets are wedge-shaped. Flowers are white or greenish and petals are rounded and barely emarginate.

Constituents: Phenolic compounds and flavonoids, particularly apigenin, apiin, and acetylapiin; essential oil, myristicin and apiol; a new monoterpene glycoside, petroside and coumarins.

Phellandrium aquaticum

Common Name: WATER DROPWORT

Family: Umbelliferae.

Habitats: Europe and Britain.

Part Used: Fruit.

Indication: Diuretic, expectorant.

Description: This plant is a biennial or perennial, having a thick, spindle-shaped root, with many whorled fibers. The stem is hollow, furrowed, half immersed in the water, very bushy, with numerous spreading, leafy branches, and from 2 to 4 feet in height. The leaves are petioled, spreading, dark-green, the flowers are white, numerous, all fertile, outer ones largest and most irregular; innermost more certainly prolific. The pedicels are shorter than the fruit.

Constituents: Ethereal oil, a yellow liquid terpene, phellandrene and alkaloids.

Phytolacca decandra

Common Names: POCK ROOT, POKEWEED

Family: Phytolaccaceae.

Habitats: America.

Part Used: Leaves.

Indication: Anti-inflammatory for swollen throat, purgative, narcotic, expell catarrh, kill sperms.

Description: This herbaceous perennial plant grows to height of 3-9 feet, stem of this plant is hollow; leaves are alternate and ovate-lanceolate, the white pinkish flowers grow with white calyx having no corolla and the fruit is a green berry that grows in clusters. It is a toxic herb with fetid foliage.

Constituents: Phytolaccatoxin and phytolaccagenin, triterpene saponins, jaligonic acid, phytolaccagenic acid (phytolaccinic acid), esculentic acid, pokeberrygenin, phytolaccasides A, B, D, E, and G, and phytolaccasaponins B, E, and G.

Pimpinella saxifraga

Common Names: BLACK CARROWAY, BURNET

Family: Umbelliferae.

Habitats: Europe.

Part Used: Roots, umbels.

Indication: Antispasmodic, astringent, carminative, diaphoretic, diuretic, stomachic.

Description: It is a perennial plant that grows from 15 to 60 cm high. The plant has a long, thick taproot with strong scent. The basal leaves are pinnate with oval and deeply serrated leaflets of different sizes and the stem leaves are alternate and of different shape.

The flowers are tiny with white, yellowish or pink petals and the seeds are small, dark brown and ovate. The plant blooms from May to September.

Constituents: Sesquiterpenoids and trinorsesquiterpene, hydrocarbons, essential oil, saponin, pimpinallin.

Pinus maritima

Common Name: SUGAR PINE

Family: Pinaceae.

Habitats: World wide.

Part Used: Sweet liquid exuded from plant.

Indication: Expectorant, laxative, bronchitis.

Description: It is a medium-size tree, reaching 20–35 m tall , bark is orange-red, leaves ('needles') are in pairs, bluish-green to distinctly yellowish-green. The cones are conic, with seeds inside, with a 20–25 mm wing, and are wind-dispersed.

Constituents: Flavonoids, catechins, pycnogenol, proanthocyanidins, and phenolic acids.

Pinus nigra

Common Name: SCOTCH PINE

Family: Pinaceae.

Habitats: Asia, and Europe.

Part Used: Leaves, stem, root, fruit, wood, gum.

Indication: Expectorant, used for inhalation in bronchitis, easing aches and pains, hair growth.

Description: It is a tree, up to 30 m tall. Bark dark gray to blackish. Young shoots glabrous. Leaves are dark green, rigid, often curved. Buds resinous. Cone ovoid, erect.

Constituents: α-pinene, ß-pinene, germacrene D, ß-caryophyllene, ß-limonene, cadinene, carene, α-terpinyl acetate, humulene, α-terpinolene, and α-muurolene and α-terpinyl acetate.

Podophyllum peltatum

Common Name: DUCK'S FOOT, WILD LEMON

Family: Berberidaceae.

Habitats: America.

Part Used: Resin of the root.

Indications: Cholagogue, antimitotic for condyloma, papilloma, warts, viral tumour.

Description: It is an indigenous, perennial herb, stem is erect, leaves are large, yellowish-green on the upper surface, paler and slightly pubescent beneath. The flower is solitary white, fragrant. The fruit is fleshy of lemon color, with brownish spots when ripe.

Constituents: Podophyllin, gum, starch, albumen, gallic acid, picropodophyllin, podophyllic acid, fixed oil, berberine and saponine .

Polygala amara

Common Name: BITTER MILK WORT

Family: Polygalaceae.

Habitats: Europe and America.

Part Used: Dried (plant) leaves.

Indication: Anti-tussive, acts on respiratory system.

Description: A perennial herb, growing to 0.2 m. It is in flower from June to August. The flowers are hermaphrodite (have both male and female organs) and are pollinated by insects. Fruits are capsular.

Constituents: Saponin, ester oligosaccharides, senegoses and methyl salicylate.

Populus alba

Common Names: QUAKING ASPEN, WHITE POPLAR

Family: Silicaceae.

Habitats: Europe, America.

Part Used: Young buds, bark, wood.

Indication: Anti-inflammatory, anti-rheumatic, balsamic, expectorant, used in hamorrhoids, heals wound and bruises.

Description: It may reach 21m or more in height and a little less than a metre in diameter. The smooth, greenish-white bark becomes dark and rough on older trees. Young green or brown twigs are coated with dense woolly hair, especially near the tip. A cross-section of the stem reveals a five-pointed, star-shaped pith. The 5 to 12 cm long leaves are oval to maple-leaf in shape with 3 to 5 broad teeth or lobes; leaves are dark green above and covered with dense white hair below. Fruits are capsular, buds are white hairy, leaves are toothed.

Constituents: Populin, salicin, a yellow coloring matter, chrysin, resin and essential oil, dipentene, glacial acetic acid, acetic ether, and amyl alcohol.

Populus trimuloides

Common Names: TREMBLING POPULAR, AMRICA ASPEN.

Family: Silicaceae.

Habitats: North Amrica, Europe.

Part Used: Bark.

Indications: Act as a nerve radish auther female catkins have one purple stigma.

Description: It is a deciduous tree having tall trunks, up to 25 m tall, with smooth pale bark, scarred with black. The glossy green leaves, dull beneath, become golden to yellow, rarely red, in autumn. The species often propagates through its roots to form large groves based on a single rhizome.

Constituents: Populin and salicin.

Pulmonaria officinalis

Common Name: LUNG WORT

Family: Boraginaceae.

Habitats: Europe.

Part Used: Flowers, leaves and shoot.

Indications: Expectorant, diuretic and astringent, help in cell regeneration, diarrhoea, haemorrhoids, throat irritation, soothe lungs, expel catarrh, cough, and bronchitis.

Description: An herbaceous, hairy perennial plant, grown as a garden flower for its drooping pink flowers that turn blue and for its often white-spotted leaves.

Constituents: Bitter astringent, mucilage.

Pulsatilla vulgaris

Common Name: WIND FLOWER, PASSE FLOWER

Family: Ranunculaceae.

Habitats: Europe.

Part Used: Leaves, flowers, stem.

Indications: Sedative and analgesic, nervous stress, spasm, headache, tension, exhaustion, otalgia, neuralgia.

Description: It is a deciduous perennial have silky, finely divided, pale green fern-like foliage that grows 10" high, with a 12" spread. Early in the spring, it produces attractive, nodding, 2"-4", primarily purple flowers with conspicuous yellow centers. The seeds are feathery with white heads.

Constituents: Potassium sulphate, amonic acid, oil of anemone.

Rheum palmatum

Common Name: RHUBARB

Family: Polygonaceae.

Habitats: China and Tibet, Asia.

Part Used: Leaves, stem, root and rhizome.

Indications: Laxative appetizer, diarrhoea, digestive stimulant, disperse blood clot, jaundice, fevers, anti-septic, anti-inflammatory, inhibit the cancer cells.

Description: It is a perennial growing to 3 m by 2 m. It is in flower from June to July, and the seeds ripen from July to September. The flowers are hermaphrodite and are pollinated by wind.

Constituents: Anthraquinones, tannins, a bitter aromatic principle.

Rhododendron ferrugineum

Common Name: SNOW ROSE/ROSEBAY.

Family: Ericaceae.

Habitats: Europe.

Part Used: Leaves and flowers.

Indication: Diuretic, anti-neuralgic, anti-rheumatic.

Description: It is bushy and evergreen shrub, height 3-5 feet, leaves are dark green, fruits are oblong capsular, seeds are flattened.

Constituents: Rhein, emodin, physcion, chrysophamol, rhaponticin, rhapontigenin, rhodxanthin, arbutin, tannins, sennosides, catechins, gallic acid, cinnaminic acid, lindleyin and oxalic acid.

Rhus aromatica

Common Names: FRAGRANT SUMACH, POISON OAK.

Family: Anacardiaceae.

Habitats: America and Canada.

Part Used: Leaves, root, bark, fruits.

Indication: Diuretic, haemmaturia, renal and urinary affection especially diabetes.

Description: It is a deciduous shrub that can grow to around 2 to 4 m tall with a rounded form. It produces yellow flowers in clusters in March or April before the leaves emerge, before anthesis. Pistillate (female) plants bear hairy red drupes in July or August that can last until the next March if not eaten by birds or small mammals. Also brewed as tea.

Constituents: Volatile and fixed oils, several resins and wax, butyric acid, tannin, glucose, gum, starch, oxalates, citric and a small quantity of malic acid.

Rhus toxicodendron

Common Name: POISON IVY

Family: Anacardiaceae.

Habitats: America.

Part Used: Fresh leaves.

Indication: Irritation of skin, eczema, vasicular erysepalas, pamphigus, inflammation of G.I.T and lungs.

Description: It grows up to a height 3 feet, stems are branched, leaves are inconsistent in shape, flowers are small, greenish white in color, fruits are globular and greyish.

Constituents: A volatile alkaloid toxicodendric acid, a non-volatile oil, toxicodendrol, wax, resin, starch, tannin (rhustannic acid).

Rosa canina

Common Name: DOG ROSE

Family: Rosaceae.

Habitat: China.

Part Used: Flower, fruit, leaves.

Indication: Revives tired eyes and skin, valued by aroma therapists.

Description: It is mainly deciduous with prickly stem.

Constituents: Flavonoids, carotenoids, fatty acids, linoleic acid, α-linolenic acid, a galactolipid, octadecatrienoyl and galactopyranosyl glycerol.

Rosmarinus officinalis

Common Name: ROSE MARY

Family: Lamiaceae.

Habitats: Asia, America.

Part Used: Flowers, leaves, shoot.

Indication: Fresh leaves and flowers are being used as a garnish, or crystallized as decoration, distilled water of flowers makes shoothing eye wash, stimulates circulation and ease aching joints by increase blood supply.

Description: It is a dense, evergreen, aromatic shrub with resinous needle like leaves, flowers are small and usually blue, also gold, silver, pink, and purple.

Constituents: A volatile oil consists of p-cymene, linalool, gamma-terpinene, thymol, beta-pinene, alpha-pinene, eucalyptol, monoterpenic hydrocarbons, oxygenated monoterpenes and sesquiterpene hydrocarbons.

Ruta graveolense

Common Name: RUE.

Family: Rutaceae.

Habitats: South africa.

Part Used: Leaves, seeds.

Indications: Leaves are rich in iron and minerals and used for tired eyes, oil has anti-sapasmodic action treats high blood pressure, also used as a stimulants.

Description: This is a evergreen sub shrub yellow summer flowers and deeply divied.

Constituents: Essential oil contains ketones, aldehydes, esters, sesquiterpene, hydrocarbons, 2-nonanone, undecanal, 2-acetoxydodecane, 2-decanone.

Salix alba

Common Name: WHITE WILLOW

Family: Salicaceae.

Habitats: Europe, West Asia.

Part Used: Leaves, shoots, wood, bark.

Indication: Stem extract is used as analgesic and febrifuge, bark extract as gargle for sore throat , and heart burn, food poisoning, leaves are used for nervous insomnia and are added to bath to ease rheumatism, root is used in leukemia and to restore bones.

Description: It is a deciduous tree growing to 25 m by 10 m at a fast rate. It is in flower from April to May, and the seeds ripen in June. The white flowers are dioecious and minute seeds are dispersed through wind.

Constituents: Salicin and tremulacin, tannin.

Salvia officinalis

Common Name: GARDEN SAGE, SAGE

Family: Lamiaceae.

Habitats: America.

Part Used: Flowers, leaves.

Indication: Anti-septic, blood tonic, flowers-as balsamic tea.

Description: It is an aromatic evergreen with grey-green textured leaves and blue flowers in summer.

Constituents: Essential oil consists of α-thujone, camphor, borneol, γ-muurolene and sclareol.

Salvia sclarea

Common Name: CLAY WORT, CLARY SAGE

Family: Lamiaceae.

Habitats: Europe and Asia.

Part Used: Flowers, leaves, seeds.

Indication: Essential oil is used for flavoring, perfumery and cosmetics, it is a powerful relaxant for stress, fatigue and menstrual disorder also in aromatherapy.

Description: It is a biennial or short-lived herbaceous perennial growing to 1 m by 0.6 m at a medium rate. It is in flower in August, and the seeds ripen in September. The blue flowers are hermaphrodite having colored bracts and large pungent leaves.

Constituents: Linalool, linalyl acetate, caryophyllene, α-terpineol, geraniol, neryl acetate, sclareol and germacrene D.

Sambucus nigra

Common Name: ELDER

Family: Adoxaceae.

Habitats: Europe and Asia.

Part Used: Flowers, leaves, shoots, fruits and root.

Indication: For cold, hay fever, sore throat, arthritis, epilepsy, mild lexative, to treat fracture and muscle spasm.

Description: It is a common, deciduous, shrub like tree. Leaves are creamy white. Flowers are white which produces wine colored berries.

Constituents: Viburnic acid,volatile oil, albumen, resin, fat, wax, tannic acid, gum, starch, pectin and various alkaline and earthy salts, an alkaloid sambucine, a glucoside sambunigrin, sugar, invertin, eldrin, an odorous oil, combined with malates of potash and lime, tyrosin.

Sanguinaria canadensis

Common Name: BLOOD WORT, RED ROOT

Family: Papaveraceae.

Habitats: Canada, America.

Part Used: Root.

Indication: Used as local anaesthetic, in chronic cough, sore throat, fever, also as anti-bacterial and anti-viral.

Description: It is a perennial, herbaceous flowering plant, rhizomes are creeping, leaves are single, large, folded at first, flowers are white.

Constituents: Sanguinarine, chelerythrine, chelirubine, sanguirubine, sanguilutine, chelilutine, the opium alkaloid protopine, and benzylisoquinoline alkaloids.

Sanguisorba officinalis

Common Names: SALAD BURNET, GREAT BURNET

Family: Rosaceae.

Habitats: Europe, North Africa, Asia.

Part Used: Flower, leaves, stem, root.

Indication: It contain Vitamin C, heals sun burns, mild diuretic, reduces tooth decay.

Description: It is a perennial growing to 1 m by 0.6 m. It is in flower from June to September. The flowers are hermaphrodite. The plant has creeping rhizome, tufts, pinnate foliage and slender stem with sphere of red tipped green blooms.

Constituents: Ziyu-Glycoside I, II, A, B, E, phenolic acid, tannin and a small amount of vitamin A.

Asplenium scolopendrium

Common Name: HART'S TONGUE FERN

Family: Polipodiáceae.

Habitats: Europe.

Part Used: Fronds.

Indications: It is astringent, cholagogue, diaphoretic, diuretic, expectorant, vulnerary. Used as an ointment in piles, burns and scalds. An infusion is taken internally for the treatment of diarrhoea, dysentery, gravelly deposits of the bladder and for removing obstructions of the liver and spleen.

Description: It is an evergreen fern growing to 0.6 m by 0.5 m at a slow rate. Plants in full sun are usually stunted and yellowish in colour, while those in full shade are dark green and luxuriant and the seeds ripen from July to August.

Rhizomes are small, scaly, reddish, fronds are erect, glossy, 30 inches long.

Constituents: An aromatic bitter substance, gallic acid mucilage, tannin.

Scrophularia nodosa

Common Name: FIGWORT, KNOTTED FIGWORT

Family: Scrophulariaceae.

Habitats: Europe.

Part Used: Flowers, leaves, shoots and roots.

Indication: Blood cleansing tonic, diuretic, stimulate heart and helps to avoid rapid heartbeat, poultice is applied for gangrene, swollen lymph glands, psoriasis, swelling, boils, small wounds.

Description: It is a perennial growing to 1 m by 0.3 m. It is in flower from June to September, and the seeds ripen from July to September. The flowers are hermaphrodite are purple brown colored, seeds are capsular round.

Constituents: Saponins, cardioactive glycosides, flavonoids, resin, sugar and organic acids.

Simarouba amara

Common Name: QUASSIA SIMAROUBA, PICRAENA OFFICINALIS

Family: Simaroubaceae.

Habitats: Madagascar, Asia (Malaysia), Australia, Mexico, Cuba, Haiti, Jamaica, and Central America.

Part Used: Leaves, bark and root.

Indication: It is antiprotozal, anti-amebic, antimalarial, and toxic to cancer and leukemia cells.

Description: It is a medium sized tree that grows up to 20 m high, with a trunk 50 to 80 cm in diameter. It produces bright green leaves 20 to 50 cm in length, small white flowers, and small red fruits. Bark-occur in flate place, yellowish or greenish color.

Constituents: Ailanthinone, benzoquinone, canthin, dehydroglaucarubinone, glaucarubine, glaucarubolone, glaucarubinone, holacanthone, melianone, simaroubidin, simarolide, simarubin, simarubolide, sitosterol, and tirucalla.

Smilax medica

Common Name: SARSAPARILLA

Family: Smilacaceae.

Habitats: Asia.

Part Used: Root, Stem, leaves.

Indications: Aphrodisiac and astringent, used in itch and ringworm, asthma, colic, cough, diabetes, reduces high blood pressure and menstrual pain.

Description: It is a toxic shrubby climber, it tastes bitter, then sweet.

Constituents: Sarsasapogenin, smilagenin, smilaxin, isoengeletin, oleanolic acid, kaempferide, dihydrokaempferide, beta-sitosterol, beta-sitosteroylglucoside, prosapogenin A sitosterol, stigmasterol, and pollinastanol; and the saponins sarsasaponin, smilasaponin, sarsaparilloside, and sitosterol glucoside.

Solanum dulcamara

Common Name: BITTER SWEET

Family: Solanaceae.

Habitats: Asia.

Part Used: Fruits, leaves, root, stem and seed.

Indications: Aphrodisiac and astringent, itch and ringworm.

Description: Vivacious plant growing from 10-20 cm high. It is shorter, finally divided leaves and flowers which are quite similar to german chamomile.

Constituents: Solanine, dulcamarin, solamin, solaceine, soladulcamarine, solarnarqenlne, solasodine, solanidine, soladulcidine, tomatidine, atropine, diosgenin, tigogenin, vamoqenln, tannins and pectin.

Solidago virgaurea

Common Name: GOLDEN ROD

Family: Asteraceae.

Habitats: Europe, North Africa and Northern, Central, and Southwestern Asia (China, Russia, India, Turkey, Kazakhstan).

Part Used: Flowers, leaves and stem.

Indications: Expectorant diuretic, mild sedative, anti-inflammatory, reduce cholesterol, treat bladder problems, fever indigestion asthma, cough, flu and sore throat.

Description: It is a perennial flowering plant. It grows in a cold climate. It grows up to 2 m. It has narrow stem. Leaves are wider with dense flowers.

Constituents: α-Pinene, myrcene, ß-pinene, limonene, sabinene, ß-germacrene-D, resin, mucilage and tannin.

Spigelia anthelmia

Common Name: PINK ROOT

Family: Loganiaceae.

Habitats: Asia and Tropical America.

Part Used: Root, whole plant.

Indications: Vermifuge, used in headaches, eye pain, and breathing difficulty.

Description: It is a perennial, grows upto 2 feet, flowers are bright red, leaves are opposite, ovate, pointed, rhizomes are dark in color, stems are herbaceous, branched, channelled.

Constituents: Spigeline, alkaloids, tannins, flavonoids, phenolic compounds, resin and volatile oil.

Steffensia elongata

Common Name: WORM SEED

Family: Piperaceae.

Habitats: North America, Europe.

Part Used: Leaves.

Indication: Anti-septic, anti-haemorrhagic.

Description: It is a tall shrub, presenting a singular appearance from the segmentary character of its stems and branches. The leaves are alternate, harsh, short-stalked, oblong-lanceolate, acuminate, pubescent beneath, tessellated or rough on the upper side on account of the sunken veins. The spikes are solitary, cylindrical and opposite the leaves; the bracts lanceolate; the flowers are bisexual, yellow, minute, and numerous. The fruit consists of small, almost black seeds.

Constituents: Maticin, an aromatic, volatile oil, nitrate of potassium, dark-green resin, artanithic acid and tannin.

Strychnos nuxvomica

Common Name: STRYCHNINE, POISON NUT

Family: Loganaiaceae.

Habitats: India, Burma, East and West Indies, South America.

Part Used: Leaves and root shrub, seed, wood.

Indication: Digestive tonic, for menstrual problems, paralysis, rabies.

Description: It is a medium-sized tree that grows in open habitats. Its leaves are ovate and 2–3.5 inches in size, flowers are greenish-white, fruits are yellow, seeds are grey.

Constituents: Strychnine, brucin.

Symphytum officinale

Common Name: COMFRAY

Family: Boraginaceae.

Habitats: United States, Europe and Western Asia.

Part Used: Leaves, bark, shoots and root.

Indication: Ulcerated digestive tract and cough renewal in damaged muscles and broken bones, poultice reduces swelling and brusing, heals cuts, burns, eczema.

Description: It is a perennial flowering plant, it has deep taproot, oval, pointed rough leaves, flowers are tubular.

Constituents: Allantoin, mucilage, steroidal saponins, tannins, pyrrolizidine alkaloids, inulin, and proteins.

Tanacetum vulgare

Common Name: TANSY TAGWORT

Family: Asteraceae.

Habitats: Europe and Asia. Naturalised in North America.

Part Used: Flowers, leaves, stem, seeds, fruits.

Indication: Powerful insect repellant, vermifuge, aerial parts are used for facial steam, also used as poultice for bruises.

Description: It is a perennial growing to 1 m by 1.5 m at a fast rate. It is in flower from August to September, and the seeds ripen from August to October. The flowers are bisexual, flowers are musted yellow, stem is erect and pungent, leaves are pinnately lobed.

Constituents: The volatile oil contains cineole, trans-thujone, camphor and myrtenol, tanacetin, tanacetotannic acid, and resin.

Taraxacum leontodon

Common Name: DANDELION

Family: Asteraceae.

Habitats: Britain and Europe.

Part Used: Root.

Indication: Diuretic, tonic and slightly aperient. It is a general stimulant to the urinary organs, and is chiefly used in kidney and liver disorders.

Description: It is weedy herb, leaves are sessile, flowers are yellow, lingulate, stems are hollow and leaf less, root is tap root.

Constituents: Taraxacin, acrystalline, an acrid resin, inulin, gluten, gum and potash.

Taxus baccata

Common Name: YEW TREE

Family: Taxaceae.

Habitat: Asia, Europe.

Part Used: Leaves and wood.

Indication: It is known for anti-cancerous qualities, particularly in treating cancers of ovaries and breast, also used in asthma, bronchitis, hiccup indigestion, rheumatism,epilepsy.

Description: It is a slow growing, long lived evergreen tree found in the wild.

Constituents: Taxin, taxicotine, milossin, tannin, tannic acid, gallic acid, volatile oil and resinous substance.

Teucrium scorodonia

Common Name: GARDEN SAGE.

Family: Lamiaceae.

Habitats: Europe and Asia.

Part Used: Leaves.

Indication: Anti-septic and anti-rheumatic.

Description: It is a perennial growing to 0.3 m by 0.5 m. It is in flower from July to September, and the seeds ripen from August to September. The flowers are bisexual. Stems are quadrangular, yellow colored flowers grow in long spikes, leaves are stalked, ovate and opposite.

Constituents: A volatile oil, some tannin and a bitter principle.

Thuja occidentalis

Common Name: ARBOR VITAE, TREE OF LIFE.

Family: Cupressaceae.

Habitats: Asia and Europe.

Part Used: Leaves, stem, bark, wood, essential oil.

Indication: Used for vaginal, urinary and bronchial infection, also used for warts and skin infections, spermatorrhea, sexual neurasthenia.

Description: It is an evergreen coniferous tree, bark is orange brown, leaves are yellow and green, shoot is upright, cones are present.

Constituents: Volatile oil, a yellow, crystallizable, bitter principle called thujin, punitannic (kowalier) and thujetic acid.

Thymus serphllum

Common Name: WILD THYME, CREEPING THYME

Family: Lamiaceae.

Habitats: Europe and Asia.

Part Used: Flowers, leaves and stem.

Indication: Used to reduced indigestion and flatulence, heals sore skin, anti-septic, calming, sedative, expectorant, cough spasm and flu.

Description: It is a subshrub growing to 2 cm tall with creeping stems up to 10 cm long. The oval evergreen leaves are 3–8 mm long. The strongly scented flowers are either lilac, pink-purple, magenta, or a rare white, produced in clusters.

Constituents: Oxygenated monoterpenes, monoterpene hydrocarbons, thymol, p-cymene, ϒ-terpinene, 1-octen-3-ol, thymol methyl ether, carvacrol methyl ether, borneol, and p-cymen-8-ol.

Tilia europaea

Common Names: LIME FLOWER, LINDEN

Family: Malvaceae.

Habitats: Europe.

Part Used: Flowers, leaves, stem and barks.

Indications: It is used for colds, cough, fever, infections, inflammation, high blood pressure, migraine, liver and gallbladder disorders and cellulitis, it is diuretic, antispasmodic and sedative.

Description: It is a deciduous broadleaf tree growing to 35 m by 15 m at a medium rate. It is in flower in July. The flowers are bisexual white or yellow in color, very small in size.

Constituents: A glucosid, tiliacin, sugar, tannin, mucilaginous matter, fatty substance, wax, yellow coloring matter, and a volatile oil.

Tussilago farfara

Common Name: COLTS FOOT

Family: Asteraceae.

Habitats: Europe, Asia and North Africa.

Part Used: Flowers, leaves and roots.

Indication: It is antitussive, astringent, demulcent, emollient, expectorant, stimulant and tonic. It is widely used in the treatment of coughs and respiratory problems, chronic emphysema and silicosis, poultice of the flowers has a soothing effect on a range of skin disorders including eczema, ulcers, sores, bites and inflammations.

Description: It is a perennial growing to 0.2 m by 1 m at a fast rate. It is in flower from February to April, and the seeds ripen from March to May. The flowers are bisexual. Rhizomes are creeping, stem is scaly, flowers are yellow.

Constituents: Mucilage, tannin, a bitter amorphous glucoside, a phytosterol and a dihydride alcohol, faradial.

Uragago ipecacuanha

Common Names: EMETIC ROOT, IPECAC ROOT

Family: Composite.

Habitats: Asia and Europe.

Part Used: Roots.

Indication: It is an emetic, used for emptying the stomach in cases of poisoning. It has also been used as a nauseant, expectorant, and diaphoretic.

Description: A low-growing tropical shrub, stem rising from 5-9 inches in height, root is cylindrical 3-4 inches in length and brown in color, leaves are oval, sessile and opposite, flowers are aggregated in solitary head having roots and rhizomes that yield emetine.

Constituents: Emetine, cephaeline, cephaelic (ipecacuanhic) acid, volatile oil, tannin.

Veronica officinalis

Common Name: SPEED WELL

Family: Plantaginaceae.

Habitats: Europe and America.

Part Used: Whole Plant.

Indication: Astringent, invigorating, appetizer and digestive expectorant diuretic and depurative, pharyngitis, catarrh, cough, bronchitis.

Description: It is a perennial herb, with ascending branches, bearing erect, spike-like clusters of blue flowers, the stems 3 to 18 inches long, leaves are opposite, shortly stalked, flowers are in dense, axillary, pale blue with dark blue stripes and bearing two stamens with a very long style. The capsule is inversely heart-shaped and notched, the entire plant is of a dull green and is generally slightly hairy, having short hairs, sometimes smooth.

Constituents: a bitter principle, an acrid principle, red colouring matter, a variety of tannic acid, producing a green colour with ferric salts, fatty acid, with malic, tartaric, citric, acetic and lactic acids; mannite; a soft, dark green bitter resin, glucosides.

Viburnum opulus

Common Names: HIGH CRANBERRY, CRAMP BARK, GUELDER ROSE

Family: Adoxaceae.

Habitats: Europe, Asia, and America.

Part Used: Stem, fruits and bark.

Indication: Sedative, anti-spasmodic, reduce muscle cramps, treat mumps by use stem bark.

Description: It is a deciduous shrub growing to 5 m by 5 m at a medium rate. It's leaves are maple like. It is in flower from June to

July, and the seeds ripen from September to October. The cream colored flowers are bisexual.

Constituents: Valerianic acid, a red coloring matter, iron-bluing tannin, and a peculiar bitter, neutral principle (viburnin), an amorphous, white substance.

Vinca minor

Common Name: LESSER PERIWINKLE

Family: Apocynaceae.

Habitats: Europe, South West Asia, America.

Part Used: Flowers, leaves and root.

Indication: Leaves are tonic and astringent and to reduced internal bleeding, menstrual bleeding ulcer and sore throat, reduced blood pressure, treat piles, nose bleeds and small wounds.

Description: It is an evergreen plant with blue, pink or white colored flowers.

Constituents: Vincamine, reserpine, reserpinine, akuammicine, majdine, vinerine, ervine, vineridine, tombozine, vincamajine, vincanine, vincanidine, vincamone, apovincamine, vincaminol, desoxyvincaminol, vincorine and perivincine.

Vincetoxicum officinale

Common Name: SWALLOW WORT

Family: Apocynaceae.

Habitats: Europe and North America.

Part Used: Leaves, foliage, flowers, seed pods and roots.

Indication: Laxative, diuretic, emetic, antitumor. Some alkaloids of the plant inhibited growth of the hormone-independent breast cancer cells.

Description: It is a perennial herb with a rhizome, stem is erect, tall and hollow, root is fibrous, leaves are opposite, short stalked, ovale, flowers are of creamy white color, fruits are elongate capsule.

Constituents: Alkaloids, C-steroid glycosides, sitosterol and triterpenoids, a-amyrin, friedelin, flavonoids and other phenolics, ß-sitosterol, stigmasterol, campestigmasterol, campesterol and hancokinol.

Viscum album

Common Names: MISTLE, MISTLETOE

Family: Santalaceae.

Habitats: Europe and Asia.

Part Used: Leaves, stems and fruits.

Indication: Heart tonic, strengthens capillary walls, stimulant to immune system, inhibits tumors.

Description: It is an evergreen shrub growing to 1 m by 1 m. It grows on the branches of other trees, to which it is attached by a swelling called a haustorium. It is in flower from February to April, and the seeds ripen from November to December. Greenish-yellow flowers are dioecious. The white berries appear from about October until May which contain single green seed.

Constituents: Flavanones, flavanone glycosides, triterpenenes, lescins, viscotoxins, choline, viscofleavin, inssosital, mannitol, saponin, salts, resin and vitamin C.

Vitis vinifera

Common Names: GRAPE, VINE

Family: Vitaceae.

Habitats: Europe and Asia.

Part Used: Leaves, stem, fruits and seeds.

Indication: It is antioxidant, antibacterial, anticancer, anti-inflammatory , antidiabetic, hepatoprotective, cardioprotective and neuroprotective.

Description: It is a deciduous climber growing to 15 m at a fast rate. It is in flower from May to July, and the seeds ripen from September to October. The leaves are alternate, palmately lobed, 5–20 cm long and broad. The flowers are bisexual. Leaves are lobed, flowers are white, yellow or pale green appear in clusters, The fruit is a berry, known as a grape; in the wild species it is 6 mm diameter and ripens light green or dark purple to blackish with a pale wax bloom.

Constituents: Phenolic compounds, anthocyanins, hydroxycinnamic acids, tannins of the proanthocyanidins type, stilbenoids, sugar, choline, carotene.

Terminology

Ablation: The separation of a component by removing the upper part, sometimes by skimming it off the surface or by wicking it up using a feather or cloth.

Albification: The making of the matter in the alchemical work become white.

Ablution: The purification of a substance by successive washings with a liquid.

Alkaloids: They mean "Alkali -like". Alkaloids are organic bases, containing Nitrogen, having specific physiological actions. Vegetable alakoids occur in any part of plants, but are generally abundant in barks, seeds, and roots.

Amalgamation: Formation of an amalgam, or alloy, of a metal with mercury. This term is sometimes extended to mean any union of metals.

Anhydrous: This term is applied to a substance, when it is completely free from water.

Ascension: When the active or subtle part rises up in the flask, usually by heating.

Assation: The reduction of a substance to a dry ash by roasting.

Bioavailablity: It is defined as the yield of the active drug from a pharmaceutical preparation at the required sites in the body.

Boiling Point: When a pure liquid boils under constant pressure and the temperature remains constant, then that constant temperature under one atmosphere sites in the body.

Calcination: The breaking down of a substance by fierce heating and burning usually in an open crucible.

Cementation: Acting upon a substance by mixing it in layers with a powdered (often corrosive) material, such as lime. This mixture is then be made to react and weld together by heating to a high temperature in a cementing furnace.

Ceration: The making of a substance to soften and appear like wax. This is often accomplished by continually adding a liquid and heating.

Cineration: The reduction of a substance to ashes by heating.

Circulation: The purification of a substance by a circular distillation in a pelican or closed distillation apparatus. Through heating the liquid component separates, is condensed and descends again to the substance in the flask.

Coadunation: Another term for coagulation.

Coagulation: The conversion of a thin liquid into a solid mixture through some inner change, as with the curdling of milk. This can be accomplished by a variety of means - by the addition of a substance, by heating or cooling.

Coction: The cooking or heating of a substance at a moderate heat for an extended period.

Colliquation: The conjuction or melting together of two fusible substances.

Coloration: Tinging a substance by adding a dye or coloured tincture. Colouring can by either by tinging the whole body or by producing a surface coating.

Combustion: The burning of a substance in the open air.

Comminution: The reduction of a substance into a powder, either by grinding, pulverising, or forcing it through a sieve.

Composition: The joining together of two different substances.

Conception: The marriage or union of the male and female aspects of substances.

Concoction: The cooking or heating of a mixture of substances at a moderate heat for an extended period.

Congelation: The conversion of a thin flowing liquid into a congealed thick substance, often by heating.

Conglutination: The conversion of a substance into a gluey mass, often by a putrefaction.

Conjunction: The joining of two opposite components, often seen as the union of the male and female, the subtle and gross, or even the elements.

Contrition: The reduction of a substance into powder only by means of fire.

Copulation: A conjunction, or joining of two opposite components, seen through the metaphor of the union of the male and female, or the union of the fixed and the volatile.

Corrosion: The eating up of a substance by an acid, alkali or corrosive material.

Cribation: The reduction of a substance to a powder by forcing through a sieve or mesh.

Crystallization: The formation of crystals out of a solution of the substance usually in water, either by their gradual formation from the liquid, or by evaporation of the liquid.

Dealbation: The making of the black substance of the alchemical process become brilliant white.

Decantation: It is a process of pouring gently and slowly a liquid (or Solution) contained in a vessel, out of a mixture of the said liquid and other insoluble solid substances, without disturbing those solid substances, which are deposited at the bottom as sediment.

Decoction: The digestion of a substance in the flask without the addition of any other material.

Decrepitation: The crackling and splitting a part of substances, for example common salt, on heating.

Deliquium: The reduction of a solid placed in a damp place to a liquid by its absorbing water from the air.

Descension: When the subtle or active part of a substance is made to go down to the bottom of a flask, rather than ascend as a vapour.

Dessication: The drying or removal of all the moisture in a substance.

Detonation: The explosive burning of substances on heating, for example substances mixed with niter.

Digestion: The slow modification of a substance by means of a gentle heat.

Disintegration: The breaking down or dissociation of a substance into different parts.

Dissociation: The breaking down or disintegration of a substance into different parts.

Dissolution: The dissolving or transforming of a substance into a liquid.

Distillation: The separation of a volatile component from a substance by heating so as to drive off the component as a vapour which is condensed and collected in a cooler part of the apparatus.

Dilution: It is method of mixing one liquid with another liquid. The more one liquid is added, the more weak the other liquid becomes in strength.

Drug: A substance which alter the function or nutrition of a part of the body. It has the capacity to effect a change in the human or animals in health or disease.

Ebullition: An effervescence produced through fermentation.

Edulceration: The washing of a salty substance till all the salts are removed.

Elaboration: The general term for the process of separating the pure from the impure, and leading a substance towards perfection, which can be done through a variety of means and processes.

Elevation: The raising of the subtle parts of a substance upwards, away from the bodily residues, into the upper parts of the vessel.

Elixeration: The conversion of a substance into an elixir.

Evaporation: The removal of the watery part of a substance by gentle heating, or being left a long time in a dry place.

Exaltation: An operation by which a substance is raised into a purer and more perfect nature.

Exhalation: The release of a gas or air from a substance.

Extraction: The preparation of the subtler and purer parts of a substance, usually by macerating it in alcohol. The extract can then be separated from the residue.

Fermentation: The rotting of a substance, usually of an organic nature, often accompanied by the release of gas bubbles.

Filtration: The process or removing the grosser parts of a substance by passing through a strainer, filter or cloth.

Fixation: The make a volatile subject fixed or solid, so that it remains permanently unaffected by fire.

Fulmination: The preparation of a fulminate or explosively unstable form of a metal. Sometimes applied to any process in which a sudden eruptive event occurs.

Fumigation: The alteration of a substance by exposing it to a corroding smoke.

Fusion: The joining of powdered substances together, or the conversion of a substance into a new form, by means of an extremely high degree of heat, sometimes using a flux.

Glutination: Turning a substance into a gluey, glutinous mass.

Gradation: The gradual purification of a substance, often through a series of stages.

Granulation: The reduction of a substance to grains or powder. There are various means of doing this - pounding, grinding, using thermal shock by heating and rapid cooling, and many others.

Grinding: The reduction of substances to a powder, usually through the use of a mortar and pestle.

Humectation: A process by which humidity is given to the substance, usually not by the direct addition of liquid, but by a gradual process of absorbing moisture.

Ignition: The self-calcination of a substance by it burning itself in a crucible.

Imbibition: The feeding of a process by the gradual and continuing addition of some substance.

Impastation: When the matter undergoing putrefaction thickens or congeals into the consistency of molten black pitch.

Impregnation: The alchemical process is sometimes paralleled with the gestation of a child. Thus impregnation follows from the union or copulation of the male and female, and leads to the generation of a new substance.

Inceration: The making of a substance into a soft waxy consistency, usually by combining it with water.

Incineration: The conversion of a substance to ashes by means of a powerful fire.

Incorporation: The mingling of mixed bodies into a conglomerate mass.

Ingression: This occurs when substances combine in such a manner that they cannot afterwards be separated.

Inhumation: To bury under the earth, sometimes used to mean any process that buries the active substance in a dark earthy material. Also applied to placing a flask in the warm heat of a dung bath.

Liquefaction: The turning of a solid material into a liquid, either by melting or dissolving.

Lixiviation: The oxidation of sulphide ores by exposing them to air and water. This forms vitriols.

Luting: The sealing of a flask or other apparatus through the use of a lute, or resinous paste which once applied sets hard and produces an airtight seal.

Maturation: A general term applied to identify the appearance of a degree of perfection in the work.

Melting: The reduction of a metal or substance to a liquid through heating.

Mortification: Here the substance undergoes a kind of death, usually through a putrefaction, and seems to have been destroyed and its active power lost, but eventually is revived.

Multiplication: The operation by which the powder of projection has its power multiplied.

Precipitation: The descent of a substance out of a solution. The precipitate descends to the bottom of the flask.

Preparation: The process by which superfluous substances are removed from the matter and that which is wanting is added to it.

Projection: The throwing of a ferment or tincture onto a substance in order to effect a transformation of the substance.

Prolectation: The separation of a substance into a subtle and more coarse part by the thinning or rarefaction of the subtler parts of the substance, rather than the coarsening of the earthy part.

Pulverisation: The breaking down of a substance to smaller fragments through being repeatedly struck with a blunt instrument, such as a hammer, or mallet.

Purgation: The purging or purifying of a substance by it casting forth a gross part.

Putrefaction: The rotting of a substance, often under a prolonged gentle moist heat. Usually the matter becomes black.

Quinta Essentia: The making of a quintessence, or highly elevated form of a substance.

Rarefaction: The making of a substance extremely subtle or thin and airy.

Rectification: The purification of the matter by means of repeated distillations, the distillate being again distilled.

Reiteration: The repetition of a process, particularly applied to circular distillation, in which the distillate is returned to the vessel, and the process continued for many cycles.

Resolution: This occurs when substances which are mixed together become violently separated by being placed into a solution. Thus milk is in this sense resolved by vinegar. This process is similar to coagulation.

Restinction: Here a substance at white heat is brought to perfection by being quenched in an exalting liquid.

Reverberation: An ignition or calcination at a high temperature, in a reverberating furnace.

Revivification: The bringing of a mortified matter back to life, or reactivating it.

Rubification: The making of the matter in the alchemical process from white to red.

Segregation: The separation of a composite substance into its parts.

Separation: The making of two opposite components separate from each other. Often alternated with the conjunction process.

Stratification: An operation which produces layers in the substance in the flask.

Subduction: The separation of abstraction downward of the subtle part, as in filtration.

Sublimation: This occurs when a solid is heated and gives off a vapour which condenses on the cool upper parts of the vessel as a solid, not going through a liquid phase. An example is sal ammoniac.

Subtilation: The separation of the subtle part of a substance from the gross.

Transudation: This occurs if the essence appears to sweat out in drops during a descending distillation.

Trituration: The reduction of a substance to a powder, not necessarily by the use of grinding, but by the application of heat.

Vitrification: The making of a substance into a glass but strong heating and sometimes the addition of lime.

Vitriolification: The making of a vitriol. Most often from a metal by the direct action of oil of vitriol, but sometimes by a more indirect route.

Appendix

A short list of key personalities of Alchemy/Spagyrics has been highlighted below:

Indian Alchemists

Kanada, Indian Sage and Philosopher, Author of Vaisheshika Sutra (6th century BC)

Nagarjuna, "Father of Latrochemistry"(150–250 CE)

Yogi Gona Vema Buddha Reddy of Nellore (25/08/1652 -?)

Arunagirinathar 15th Century Sage and Philosopher

Vallalar, 18th Century Sage and Philosopher

Chinese Alchemists

Wei Boyang Chinese alchemist of the Eastern Han Dynasty (ca.142CE)

Zhang Guo the Elder (c. 600) Chinese alchemist of the Tang Dynasty

Arabian Alchemists

Geber (Abu Musa Jabir Ibn Hayyan) (721-815 AD)

Geber (Abu Musa Jabir Ibn Hayyan) (721-815 AD)

Khalid ibn Yazid, "Calid" (d. 704)

Jbir ibn Hayyn, "Geber" (c. 721-815)

Dhul-Nun al-Misri (b. 796)

Muhammad ibn Zakar+ya Rzi, "Rhazes" (864-930)

Muhammed ibn Umail al-Tamimi, "Senior Zadith" (c. 900-960)

Al-Farabi, "Alfarabi" (870-950/951)

Ibn Sina or Avicenna (980-1037)

European Alchemists

Maria Prophetissima or Mary the Jewess (ca.300CE)

Cleopatra the Alchemist (Cleopatra the Alchemist) (c.-350-c.-300)

Hypatia of Alexandria (350-370 to 415 AD)

Alain de Lille (1128-1202)

Al-Tughrai (1061-1121)

Artephius (c. 1150)

Albertus Magnus (1193-1280)

Roger Bacon (1214-1294)

Nicholas & Perenelle Flamel (ca 1330-1418CE)

Pseudo-Geber (Spain, 13th century)

Ramon Llull (1232-1315)

Arnold of Villanova (1245 – ?(before 1311))

Pope John XXII (1249-1334)

John Dastin (early 14th)

Gilles de Rais (1404-1440)

Bernard Trevisan (1406-1490)

George Ripley (1802-1880)

Thomas Norton (1532-1584)

Johannes Trithemius (1462-1516)

Heinrich Cornelius Agrippa (1486-1535)

Paracelsus (Philippus Aureolus Theophrastus Bombastus von Hohenheim)(1493-1541)

Basilius Valentinus 15th Century German Alchemist

John Dee (1527-1609)

Edward Kelley (1555-1597)

Johann Georg Faust (1480-1540)

François Hotman (1524-1590)

Tycho Brahe (1546-1601)

Heinrich Khunrath (1560-1605)

Michael (1568-1622)

Jan Baptist van Helmont (1580-1644)

Arthur Dee (1579-1651)

Edward Dyer (1543-1607)

Elias Ashmole (1617-1692)

Johann Friedrich Schweitzer (1625-1709)

George Starkey (1628-1665)

Claude Duval (1643-1670)

Robert Boyle (1627-1691)

Hennig Brandt (ca. 1630-1710)

Isaac Newton (1643-1727)

Edmund Dickinson (1624-1707)

Alessandro Cagliostro (1743-1795)

Count of St. Germain (1712-1784)

Count Cesare Mattei (1809-1896)

Carl Friedrich Zimpel (1801-1879)

Johann Conrad Glückselig (1864-1934)

Theodor Krauss (1884-1924)

Demeter Georgievitz-Weitzer (1873-1949)

Alexander von Bernus (1880-1965)

Ernest Rutherford (1871-1937)

August Strindberg (1849-1912)

Franz Tausend (1884-1942)

Fulcanelli (1839-1953)

Frater Albertus (1911-1984)

Bibliography

1. Hans Nintzel - "Alchemy" (article in The Complete Golden Dawn System of Magic, Israel Regardie, Falcon Press, 1984. Part 2; pp. 52-61).
2. Alex Sumner - Herbal Alchemy on a Budget (Journal of the Western Mystery Tradition, No. 9, Vol. 1, Autumnal Equinox 2005).
3. Healing Codes For The Biological Apocalypse by Dr. Leonard Horowitz.
4. Rattemeyer M., Popp F. A., Nagl, W. (1981) Evidence of photon emission from DNA in living systems, Nature Wissenshanften, 68 (11): 572-573.
5. The Quest for the Secret Force of the Universe, by Lynne McTaggart.
6. Boyd L J. A Study of the Simile in Medicine. Philadelphia: Boericke and Tafel, 1936.
7. Behring E. Gesammelte Abhandlungen. Neue Folge. Bonn: Marcus and Weber, 1915.
8. Bellavite P, Signorini A. The Emerging Science of Homeopathy. Berkeley, CA: North Atlantic Books, 2002.
9. Coulter H. : Divided Legacy, vol. II. The Origins of Modern Western Medicine: J.B. van Helmont to Claude Bernard. Berkeley, CA: North Atlantic Books, 1977.
10. Coulter H. : Divided Legacy, vol. I. The Patterns Emerge, Hippocrates to Paracelsus. Washington: Center for Empirical Medicine, 1975.
11. Lux W. Isopathie der Contagionen. Liepzig: Ed Kollmann, 1833.

12. Griesselich L. Handbuch zur kenntnis der homoeopatischen oder specifischen heilkunst. Karlsruhe: Malsch und Vogel, 1848.
13. Reckeweg HH. Homotoxikologie. Ganzheitsschau Einer Synthese der Medizin. Baden-Baden: Aurelia Verlag, 1981.
14. Prof. Mario Facci, Count Cesare Mattei Lord of Rocchetta in History and Medicine (2014).
15. Schulz H. Uber die Theorie der Arzneimittelwirkung. Virchows Arch 1877;108:423–34.
16. Schulz H. Uber Hefegifte. Arch Fuer Physiol 1888;42:517–41.
17. Martius F. Das Arndt-Schulz Grundgesetz. Muench Med Wschr 1923;70: 1005–6.
18. Linde K, ter Riet G, Hondras M, Melchart D, Willich SN. Characteristics and quality of systematic reviews of acupuncture, herbal medicines, and homeopathy. Forsch Komplementarmed Klass Naturheilkd 2003;10: 88–94.
19. Bernus, A. v.: alchemy and healing arts, publishing at the Goetheanum.
20. Burckhardt, T.: alchemy - meaning and the world, Dingfelder-Verlag.
21. Frater Albertus: The Alchemist of the Rocky Mountains, Alpha and Omega GmbH.
22. Fritschi, HJ: Spagyrik—Academic and Working Paper, Gustav Fischer Verlag.
23. Gebelein, H.: alchemy, Diederichs-Verlag.
24. Gilchrist, Ch: Alchemy, Aurum-Verlag.
25. Grohmann, F.: Healthy through alchemy, Freya-Verlag.
26. Haage, BD: Alchemy in the Middle Ages, Artemis-Verlag.
27. Helmrich, H.: Spagyrik, Haug-Verlag.
28. Junius, M. : Practical Handbook of Plant alchemy, Ansata-Verlag.

29. Ulrich Arndt: The Mastery of Spagyric Medicine, Innovative Medicine, LLC., Nov, 2012.

30. Hans-Josef Fritschi: "Spagyric, Lehr- und Arbeitsbuch", Gustav Fischer verlag. Ulm 1997.

31. Helmut Gebelein: "Alchemie, Die Magie des Stofflichen", Diedrichs Verlag, Munich, 1996.

32. Alexander Roob: "Alchemie und Mystik", Bendikt Taschen Verlag, Colonge, 1996.

33. Rudolf Hauscka: "Substanzlehre", Klostermann GmbH, Frankfurt, 1990.

34. Peter Schleicher: "Grundzuge der Immundiagnostik und Immuntherapie", Hippokrates Verlag, Stuttgart, 1997.

35. Köster, P.: Spagyrik, Die Alternative: Heilung aus Pflanzen. München: EhrenwirtVerlag 1991.

36. Encyclopaedia of Indian Medicine Historical perspective by Saligrama Krishna Ramachandra Rao, Popular Prakashan, Mumbai, 1985.

37. Natural Medicines by Dr. Debasish Kundu & Dr. Malik A.K. Awan (Kruger Brentt, U.K.).

38. Bolton, Dr.H.Carrington : Iatro-chemistry, Science Journal, Vol. VII, No. 169 (March 25, 1898).

39. Whitmont, E.: The alchemy of healing, Burgdorf-Verlag.

40. Kundu Debasish : Spagyric Medicine: Purification of Body, Mind and Spirit, Alternative and Integrative Medicine Journal, October, 2013.

41. Kundu Debasish : Alchemy from Mystery to Medicine, Homoeopathic Links, Issue 02, Volume 27, June 2014.

42. Kundu Sudeshna and Debasish: Count Cesare Mattei's Liquid Color Therapy, International Journal of Homeopathy and Natural Medicines, Issue 3, Volume 1, October 2015, Pages: 28-34.

Recommended Further Reading:

1. Kundu Debasish, Ahmed M, Jayasuriya A: Materia Medica for the New Age Man (Originals, 2016).
2. Kundu Debasish, Sin Choo Led: Essentials of Acupuncture (Originals, 2017).
3. Kundu Debasish: Notes on Spagyrics (Originals, 2017).
4. Kundu Debasish, Agnihotri Vijai Kant, Pezzani Raffaele : A Treatise on Spagyric Homoeopathic Pharmacy (Originals, 2017).
5. Kundu Debasish: Mysticism, Romance & Secrets of Count Cesare Mattei (LBO Publishing, USA, 2017).